T025988

06. JUL 12,

D1628485

QV 474
03/12

OF01032

An Insider's Guide to Clinical Trials

Curtis L. Meinert

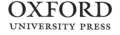

OXFORD
UNIVERSITY PRESS

OXFORD
UNIVERSITY PRESS

Oxford University Press, Inc., publishes works that further
Oxford University's objective of excellence
in research, scholarship, and education.

Oxford New York
Auckland   Cape Town   Dar es Salaam   Hong Kong   Karachi
Kuala Lumpur   Madrid   Melbourne   Mexico City   Nairobi
New Delhi   Shanghai   Taipei   Toronto

With offices in
Argentina   Austria   Brazil   Chile   Czech Republic   France   Greece
Guatemala   Hungary   Italy   Japan   Poland   Portugal   Singapore
South Korea   Switzerland   Thailand   Turkey   Ukraine   Vietnam

Copyright © 2011 by Oxford University Press, Inc.

Published by Oxford University Press, Inc.
198 Madison Avenue, New York, New York 10016
www.oup.com

Library of Congress Cataloging-in-Publication Data

Meinert, Curtis L.
An insider's guide to clinical trials/Curtis L. Meinert.
    p.; cm.
Includes bibliographical references and index.
ISBN 978-0-19-974296-7 (pbk.: alk. paper)
1. Clinical trials. I.   Title.
[DNLM: 1.   Clinical Trials, Phase III as Topic—United States.
2.   Clinical Trials, Phase IV as Topic—United States.
3.   Randomized Controlled Trials as Topic—United States. QV 771]
R853.C55M43 2011
610.72'4—dc22   2010027745
ISBN-13: 9780199742967

9 8 7 6 5 4 3 2 1
Printed in USA
on acid-free paper

To my daughters Julie, Nancy, and Jill
and
my grandchildren Edward, Matthew, Rachael, and Allison.

Acknowledgments

One cannot write a book without encouragement and help—lots of it. My help came from having an understanding wife, **Susie**, who tolerates the orneriness and messes book writing generates. Thank you!

It comes also from **Betty Collison** (Watson)—my right hand at work. She has been a masterful "reader," "checker," and "getter."

Help from **Susan Tonasica**, a faculty member in the Department of Epidemiology here at Hopkins, has been constant since my coming to Hopkins in 1980; for this work as a reader and editor.

Early on in this effort, I recruited a cadre of people with varying knowledge of clinical trials. Their job was to read PDF versions of chapters as they were produced and to provide feedback. That cadre was:

My wife

My three daughters, **Julie Meinert Smith** (Hair Stylist, Manassas, Virginia), **Nancy Meinert Courduff** (Nutritionist, Baltimore), and **Jill Meinert** (Programmer, Johns Hopkins, Baltimore)

Betty Collison (Senior Administrative Coordinator, Johns Hopkins)

Stacie Reiner Johnson (CPA, Minneapolis)

Beth Kaping (R.N., Certified Clinical Research Coordinator, Mayo Clinic)

John Matson (Veterinarian [retired], Des Moines)

Lee McCaffrey (Senior Research Associate, Johns Hopkins)
Kendra Meinert (Journalist, Green Bay)
Cynthia Regnier (Lead R.N. Study Coordinator, Mayo Clinic)
Susan Tonascia (Senior Scientist, Johns Hopkins)
Thanks to all of them!

Jill Meinert deserves special mention. Being the family geek, she has patiently, and always with good grace, helped me through the electronic messes one stumbles into with things like book writing. She has generated many of the PubMed counts scattered throughout the book and has produced line sketches featured in various chapters of the book.

Thanks to **Joan Bossert** (Editor, Oxford University Press) for her guidance, support, and her wisdom. She is the best!

Other thanks to:

Betty Collison for her work sketching 2006 trials referenced in Chapters 5, 6, and 23

Ann Ervin (Assistant Scientist, Johns Hopkins) for help in tracking down various systematic reviews and meta-analyses

Jill Meinert for entry of data and analyses of data used in Chapters 5, 6, and 23.

Mark Van Natta (Senior Statistician, Johns Hopkins) for help in analyses included in Chapter 17.

Bonnie and **Steve Piantadosi** (formerly at Johns Hopkins, now in Los Angeles, where Steve is Director of the Samuel Oschin Comprehensive Cancer Institute of Cedars-Sinai) for their encouragement.

Contents

Preface

Never try to teach a pig how to sing. It wastes your time and annoys the pig.

Robert Heinlein

My career as a trialist was an accident.

I was working on my Ph.D. dissertation when Chris Klimt arrived at the University of Minnesota in 1960, looking for someone to help in the design and execution of a multicenter trial—the University Group Diabetes Program. Word came that he wanted to interview several "almost finished" students in biostatistics, me among them.

But I had zero interest in signing on with anyone until I finished my dissertation, so I ignored the invitation, until my advisor got on my case. Not wishing to be rude, I went for the interview—and signed on.

Another university and several trials later, I got the book writing bug. I aspired to write a textbook on the design and conduct of clinical trials. The bug was serious enough to cause me to take a sabbatical from the University of Maryland to jump-start the effort. But, after six months of staring at blank pages, I had purged myself of the bug.

Then, a university later, when I moved across town to Johns Hopkins and into the Department of Epidemiology in the School of Public Health in 1980, the bug hit again. It was incubated by the job of creating and teaching an introductory course on clinical trials to medical and graduate students. I got rid of it in 1986, by finishing the book I had abandoned years back.

Years of teaching and working with groups doing trials have driven home the point that trials are deceptively simple: State a question, find some patients, randomize them to treatment, collect some data, analyze the data, write up the results, and move on.

How hard can it be to teach people that? I got my first lesson teaching my father.

Every year, after moving to Baltimore, we would travel back to Minnesota to visit my parents. On various occasions, my father would ask what I did. Every time he asked, I tried to explain. Every time, after I finished, it would be obvious that he did not understand how I could get paid for doing nothing.

On our last visit, shortly before he died, he asked again, so I tried again. His eyes got glassy, but being an experienced classroom teacher, I pressed on.

When I finished, he leaned back in his chair and said, "It sounds to me like you sit around in a white shirt and tie, feet up on the desk, and talk smart." I said, "I guess that's about it," and moved on to another topic.

Being a trialist and, therefore, a "show me the evidence" type, has its domestic problems, seeing as I live with a wife who needs "less evidence" than her husband. Years ago, she decided that our mostly house dog Cheb (named after the Russian mathematician Pafnuty Chebyshev) should go on heartworm medication. I said, "Show me the evidence that the benefits outweigh the risks." "You and your evidence!," she snapped. Our marriage survived, but Cheb went on heartworm medication. So much for evidence when your mind is made up.

But, in spite of that setback and many others on the "evidence front," my wife is the reason for this book. It was obvious, after years of interaction, that she has a genuine interest in trials and in what they teach us about what is good and bad for us. But it was obvious to me that I was not going to make her into a trialist. She was interested in trials, but not interested enough to read a textbook on how they are designed and conducted.

Those interactions and hundreds of teaching experiences have served as the driving force behind this book.

The *Guide* is intended for students and professionals or researchers not familiar with clinical trials. The focus is on randomized phase III and

IV trials. My aim has been to offer insights into the workings of trials from the inside, in the hope of making the learning curve for aspiring trialists more gentle. This aim explains the sometime-colloquial approach to discourse. Having taught introductory courses in clinical trials for years with more sleepers than Motel 6, I am painfully aware that the basics of trials can be as interesting as watching paint dry. Hence, in this effort, I decided to lighten up with touches of "down home" writing in the hope of empty rooms at Motel 6.

CLM
Towson, Maryland
June 2010
An Insider's Guide to Clinical Trials

And further, by these, my son, be admonished: Of making many books there is no end; and much study is a weariness of the flesh.

Ecclesiastes 12:12

1

Introduction

Progress: Making new mistakes

CLM

*T*rial is of Anglo-French origin, meaning to choose, sort, select, or try. *Clinical* is of French and Greek origin, pertaining to the practice of medicine (feminine of *klinikos*, from *klinē*, meaning couch or bed for the sick). Hence, *clinical trial* literally refers to the trying of something on people in sick beds to determine if that something works. More prosaically, a clinical trial is an experiment done on people to determine if a treatment is safe and effective, whether or not they are on their sick beds. Indeed, a fair number of trials are done on well people in an effort to prevent illness. As a matter of fact, the largest trial ever done involved well people and mostly children: the polio vaccine trial, which started in 1954 and concluded a year later. Done to test the safety and efficacy of the Salk vaccine, the trial involved upward of 2 million children.[49, 76]

The modifier *clinical*, is used to denote the fact that the "trying" or "testing" is done on humans, in vivo or in vitro. Strictly speaking, its use should be limited to "trying" done on humans in the "sick bed," but often is retained even in references to trials done on healthy people, for example, as in references to primary prevention trials.

In everyday usage, the term *clinical trial* can refer to an uncontrolled experiment involving just one or two people or to a controlled experiment involving thousands of people. *Controlled*, as used herein, means the experiment is "internally comparative," as discussed in Chapter 3.

The treatment unit in in-vivo trials may be persons, aggregates of persons (e.g., members of a household or larger aggregates, such as entire villages), or parts of persons (e.g., a person's eyes or hands). The treatment unit may receive two or more of the study treatments in some sequence (e.g., as in *crossover trials*) or one and only one of the study treatments (e.g., as in *parallel-treatment trials*). The treatment or sequence of treatments may be arbitrarily selected or determined by randomization. The focus here is on randomized parallel-treatment trials.

The notion of "trying" to determine effectiveness is not new. The Book of Daniel (1:12–15) contains an account of a diet trial:

> Prove thy servants, I beseech thee, ten days; and let them give us pulse to eat, and water to drink. Then let our countenances be looked upon before thee, and the countenance of the children that eat of the portion of the King's meat: and as thou seest, deal with thy servants. So he consented to them in this matter, and proved them ten days. And at the end of ten days their countenances appeared fairer and fatter in flesh than all the children which did eat the portion of the King's meat. (American Bible Society, 1816).[5]

One of the earliest trials having a concurrently enrolled and treated control group was done by a Scottish-educated surgeon, James Lind (1716–1794), while on board the HMS *Salisbury* at sea. He was trying to find a treatment for a common condition among sailors on ships on long sea voyages—scurvy.

> On the 20th of May 1747, I took twelve patients in the scurvy, on board the Salisbury at sea. Their cases were as similar as I could have them. They all in general had putrid gums, the spots and lassitude, with weakness of their knees. They lay together in one place, being a proper apartment for the sick in the fore-hold; and had one diet common to all, viz., watergruel sweetened with sugar in the morning; fresh mutton-broth often times for dinner; at other times puddings, boiled biscuit with sugar, etc; and for supper, barley and raisins, rice and currants, sago and wine, or the like. Two of these were

ordered each a quart of cyder a day. Two others took twenty-five gutts of elixir vitriol three times a day, upon an empty stomach; using a gargle strongly acidulated with it for their mouths. Two others took two spoonfuls of vinegar three times a day, upon an empty stomach; having their gruels and their other food well acidulated with it, as also the gargle for their mouth. Two of the worst patients, with the tendons in the ham rigid (a symptom none of the rest had), were put under a course of seawater. Of this they drank half a pint every day, and sometimes more or less as it operated, by way of gentle physic. Two others had each two oranges and one lemon given them every day. These they eat with greediness, at different times, upon an empty stomach. They continued but six days under this course, having consumed the quantity that could be spared. The two remaining patients, took the bigness of a nutmeg three times a-day, of an electuary recommended by an hospital surgeon, made of garlic, mustard-seed, rad raphan, balsam of Peru, and gum myrrh; using for common drink, barley-water well acidulated with tamarinds; by a decoction of which, with the addition of cremor tartar, they were gently purged three or four times during the course.

Those receiving a daily ration of oranges and lemons fared best.

The consequence was, that the most sudden and visible good effects were perceived from the use of the oranges and lemons; one of those who had taken them, being at the end of six days fit for duty.[74]

Despite these results, Lind and many others at the time still clung to the notion that the best treatment involved placing patients stricken with scurvy in "pure dry air." The reluctance to accept oranges and lemons as treatment for the disease had to do, in part, with the relative expense of acquiring such fruits. We think they grow in supermarkets today, but back then it was a different story. The "treatment" was expensive. It was 1795 before the British Navy supplied lemon and lime juice for its ships at sea,[39] hence paving the way for British sailors to be known as "limeys."

The concept of *randomization* as a device for treatment assignment was introduced by Fisher, while he was involved in agricultural experimentation.[18,44-46] Amberson and his coworkers[4], in a study of sanocrysin in the treatment of pulmonary tuberculosis published in 1931, were among the first to use randomization for treatment assignment in an actual clinical trial.

Table 1.1 Lind's design

Sample size
   Total..12
   Per treatment group...2

No. of treatments 6

Test treatments...5
   Cyder, 1 qt/day
   Elixir vitriol, 25 gutts, 3 times/day
   Vinegar, 2 spoonfuls, 3 times/day
   Oranges (2); lemon (1)/day
   Bigness of nutmeg 3 times/day
Control treatment...1
   Sea-water, 1/2 pt/day

Length of follow-up ....6 days

Outcome measure ....Fitness for duty

The 24 patients were then divided into two approximately comparable
groups of 12 each. The cases were individually matched, one with another,
in making this division . . . Then, by a flip of the coin, one group became
identified as group I (sanocrysin-treated) and the other as group II (control).
The members of the separate groups were known only to the nurse in charge
of the ward and to two of us. The patients themselves were not aware of any
distinctions in the treatment administered.

It would be several years later before randomization was used for
assigning individuals to treatment. Diehl and co-workers (1938)[37] described
a method of randomly assigning University of Minnesota student volun-
teers to treatment in a double-masked, placebo-controlled trial involving
treatment of the common cold.

Sir Austin Bradford Hill is widely regarded as the father of modern clinical trial design, and he, among others, was a leading force in the development of modern-day clinical trials. Hill's 1962 book *Statistical Methods in Clinical and Preventive Medicine*[59] represented an important milestone in the field of clinical trials.

The Medical Research Council of the United Kingdom established a committee in 1931 to promote and assist in the development of clinical trials:

> The Medical Research Council announce that they have appointed a Therapeutic Trials Committee, as follows, to advise and assist them in arranging for properly controlled clinical tests of new products that seem likely, on experimental grounds, to have value in the treatment of disease. . . . The Therapeutic Trials Committee will be prepared to consider applications by commercial firms for the examination of new products, submitted with the available experimental evidence of their value, and appropriate clinical trials will be arranged in suitable cases.[78] (Medical Research Council, 1931)

The concept of multiple investigators from different sites, all following a common study protocol in the conduct of a clinical trial, did not emerge until the late 1930s and early 1940s. One of the first applications of this approach was reported in a 1944 publication of a trial to evaluate patulin for treatment of the common cold.[103]

A multicenter trial involving the use of streptomycin in patients with pulmonary tuberculosis was published in 1948.[77] One of the first multicenter trials in the United States involved assessment of the same drug.[88–90] The study was initiated at about the same time as the British study, but it did not produce any published results until 1952, four years after the British publication.

The Veterans Administration (VA), in conjunction with the United States Armed Services, carried out a series of multicenter trials between 1945 and 1960 in an attempt to establish the efficacy of various chemotherapeutic agents in the treatment of tuberculosis.[118] The VA provided support for various other multicenter trials in the 1960s, under a relatively informal funding structure. A more formal structure was created in 1972.

The creation of the National Cancer Institute in 1937 signaled the start of federally sponsored medical research in the United States and the creation of what ultimately has come to constitute the National Institutes of Health.[96] The Institutes of this agency support by far the largest number of trials among all U.S. governmental agencies. The largest and most complex multicenter trials have been carried out by the National Heart, Lung, and Blood Institute (NHLBI). Some, such as the Multiple Risk Factor Intervention Trial and the Hypertension Detection and Follow-Up Program,[91] have involved thousands of patients and years of follow-up.[61]

One of the first multicenter trials sponsored by the National Heart Institute (now the NHLBI) was a trial involving the use of adrenocorticotropin hormone (ACTH), cortisone, and aspirin as a treatment for rheumatic heart disease. The trial was initiated in 1951 and was carried out in conjunction with the Medical Research Council of Great Britain, the American Heart Association, and the Canadian Arthritis and Rheumatism Society.[111]

Multicenter trials focusing on the treatment of chronic noninfectious diseases began to appear in the 1960s. One of the first examples in this category was the University Group Diabetes Program, started in 1960 and completed in 1974.[123,126] The advent of such trials has served to stimulate communication across disciplines, as evidenced by the formation of the Society for Clinical Trials in 1979, and publication of *Controlled Clinical Trials* starting in 1980.[80]

By the late 1960s, multicenter trials were regarded as the "indispensable ordeal" by Donald Fredrickson (Director of the National Heart Institute, 1966–1968 and Director of the NIH, 1975–1981) in an address before the New York Academy of Science in 1968:

> Field trials are indispensable. They will continue to be an ordeal. They lack glamor, they strain our resources and patience, and they protract the moment of truth to excruciating limits. Still, they are among the most challenging tests of our skills. I have no doubt that when the problem is well chosen, the study is appropriately designed, and that when all the populations concerned are made aware of the route and the goal, the reward can be commensurate with the effort. If, in major medical dilemmas, the alternative is to pay the cost of perpetual uncertainty, have we really any choice?

A major stimulus for clinical trials came in 1962, from the U.S. Congress, in the form of the Kefauver-Harris amendment to the Food,

Drug, and Cosmetic Act of 1938. The amendment set forth a series of requirements that had to be satisfied before a drug could be approved for marketing by the Food and Drug Administration (FDA).[24,47,69,120] The amendment spelled out the nature of scientific evidence required for a drug approval—a specification heavily dependent on what are referred to in the Act as "adequate and well-controlled investigations."

The term "substantial evidence" means evidence consisting of adequate and well-controlled investigations, including clinical investigations, by experts qualified by scientific training and experience to evaluate the effectiveness of the drug involved, on the basis of which it could fairly and responsibly be concluded by such experts that the drug will have the effect it purports or is represented to have under the conditions of its use prescribed, recommended, or suggested in the labeling or proposed labeling thereof.[120]

Trials are externally or internally comparative. Lind's trial was internally comparative. Trials are internally comparative if they:

1. Involve two or more treatment regimens/groups for comparison
2. Have explicit enrollment criteria
3. Have explicit landmarks defining the point of enrollment
4. Involve concurrent enrollment, treatment, and follow-up of the people represented in the different treatment groups

There is nothing to compare internally absent the first condition. There is no way of defining the study population absent condition 2 and 3, and the comparison is suspect absent condition 4.

Absent these four requirements, trials, by default, are externally comparative. The trial described in the Book of Daniel is externally comparative by virtue of the fact that it lacked requirements 2 and 3.

The National Library of Medicine (NLM) definition of clinical trial is:

Work that is the report of a pre-planned clinical study of the safety, efficacy, or optimum dosage schedule of one or more diagnostic, therapeutic, or prophylactic drugs, devices, or techniques in humans selected according to predetermined criteria of eligibility and observed for predefined evidence of favorable and unfavorable effects.

The definition is purposely broad to capture internally as well as externally comparative trials. If the focus is on comparative trials, one has to search the NLM database for "randomized controlled trial":

> Work consisting of a clinical trial that involves at least one test treatment and one control treatment, concurrent enrollment and follow-up of the test- and control-treated groups, and in which the treatments to be administered are selected by a random process, such as the use of a random-numbers table.

Trials that are externally comparative rely on *historical controls* (or *literature controls*) for comparison. A historical comparison group is a collection of people having had the disease or condition being treated in the trial at hand, but in an earlier, nonconcurrent time before the treatment being tested was available and who are hence free of exposure to the treatment at issue. Use is limited to diseases having a well-known course. If the new treatment is seen as markedly altering that course, it is argued that the treatment represents an advance and hence should be used.

But the reality is that the road to hell is paved with historical controls because: (a) the natural history is rarely that well known; (b) of the opportunity to pick controls that maximize the difference; (c) of artifactual effects related simply to the temporal difference represented; and (d) there is no way to know whether the two groups are comparable with regard to factors that may influence outcome.

It is difficult enough to draw conclusions regarding the merits of a treatment when a concurrent comparison group exists. It is treacherous indeed when lacking such a group.

Single- vs. Multicenter Trials

Trials are either single-center or multicenter.

> **single-center trial** - A trial done at a single site: (a) Such a trial, even if performed in association with a coalition of clinics in which each clinic performs its own trial; (b) A trial not having any clinical centers and a single resource center, e.g., the Physicians' Health Study.[105] Ant: multicenter trial

multicenter trial - 1. A trial involving two or more clinical centers, a common study protocol, and a data center, data coordinating center, or coordinating center to receive, process, and analyze study data. 2. A trial involving at least one clinical center and one or more resource centers. Syn: collaborative trial, cooperative trial ant: single-center trial.

Trials default to being multicenter when it is a practical impossibility to enroll the numbers required at a single center in any reasonable time period. For example, the Women's Health Initiative (WHI) primary prevention trial in postmenopausal women comparing estrogen plus progestin versus placebo involved 16,600 women followed at 40 clinics.[130] Incidentally, the results of that trial—results suggesting that "overall health risks exceeded benefits from use of combined estrogen plus progestin"—underscore why observational data cannot be relied on as the sole indicator of the benefits of a treatment. The observational studies available when the trial was designed in the early 1990s suggested that estrogen replacement in postmenopausal women reduced the risk of coronary heart disease. For example, Stampfer and Colditz concluded, after review of data from 16 prospective observational studies, that "the bulk of the evidence strongly supports a protective effect of estrogens that is unlikely to be explained by confounding factors."[115]

Trials are also sometimes characterized by phase, especially in relation to a new drug, in the FDA sense of "new" (see Chapter 3):

- **phase I trial**—A trial involving the first applications of a new treatment to human beings; conducted to generate preliminary information on safety; usually uncontrolled.
- **phase II trial**—A trial involving a second stage of testing of a new treatment in human beings; done to generate preliminary information on efficacy and added information on safety; may or may not be randomized.
- **phase III trial**—A randomized controlled trial of a largely heretofore untested treatment intended primarily to generate information on efficacy as measured against a control treatment; for drugs done under an Investigational New Drug (IND), the final stage in testing before licensure.

- **phase IV trial**—A randomized controlled trial involving a clinical event as the primary outcome measure and providing for extended treatment (when appropriate) and long-term follow-up, with efficacy and safety of the treatment being measured against a designated control treatment; when in reference to drug trials involving licensed drugs.

Classification of Trials by Design

Trials can also be classified by the nature of the treatment design:

- **parallel-treatment design**—A treatment design in which persons are assigned to receive one and only one of the study treatments; hence, one in which treatment groups are comprised of different persons.
- **crossover treatment design**—A treatment design that provides for the administration of two or more of the study treatments, one after another, in a specified or random order, to persons; each administration may be followed by a *washout period* (the period of time separating the last administration of a treatment in one period and the first administration of a new one in the next period; necessary for body to clear the effect of the previous treatment before administering the new treatment); hence, one in which treatment groups are comprised of the same people.

The majority of trials published involve parallel-treatment designs. Most crossover trials involve short periods of treatment, and comparisons are based on changes in some laboratory measure.

2

The Language of Clinical Trials

It is the fate of those who toil at the lower employments of life, to be rather driven by the fear of evil, than attracted by the prospect of good; to be exposed to censure, without hope of praise; to be disgraced by miscarriage, or punished for neglect, where success would have been without applause, and diligence without reward.

Among these unhappy mortals is the writer of dictionaries; whom mankind have considered, not as the pupil, but the slave of science, the pioneer of literature, doomed only to remove rubbish and clear obstructions from the paths of Learning and Genius, who press forward to conquest and glory, without bestowing a smile on the humble drudge that facilitates their progress. Every other author may aspire to praise; the lexicographer can only hope to escape reproach, and even this negative recompense has been yet granted to very few.

Preface to *A Dictionary of the English Language*, Samuel Johnson, 1755.[67]

As a literalist, I panicked the first time I pulled into Union Station in Washington, D.C., when the conductor announced "All doors will not open." "How the hell am I going to get out of here?" I mused, as I prepared to kick out a window, only to discover that he meant "only some doors will open."

Similarly, I have always wondered what airline flight attendants meant when they said "No smoking is permitted." Did they mean one should not smoke or that it was OK to not smoke?

Likewise, as a trialist, every time I hear mention of "placebo patients" I wonder how they managed to get them sugar-coated. Such is the baggage of a dictionary writer.[83]

As with any field, trialists have their own lexicon. Hence, "a once lightly through the tulip patch" of "clinical trials speak" is indicated.

Randomization

Randomization as a noun is (1) The act of assigning or ordering that is the result of a random process such as that represented by a sequence of numbers in a table of random numbers or a sequence of numbers produced by a random number generator, e.g., the assignment of a patient to treatment using a random process. (2) The process of deriving an order or sequence of items, specimens, records, or the like using a random process.

Randomization, random, and *randomized* are currency words in the art form of comparative trials. Mere mention of them in relation to the process of assigning persons to treatment confers an aura of respectability to the trial. That being so, there is the ever-present temptation to use them simply to garner luster. Part of the misuse comes from the fact that *random,* as an adjective in lay usage, refers to a process having or appearing to have no specific pattern, course, or objective and is used interchangeably with haphazard. But *random,* as an adjective in scientific discourse, refers to a process producing a sequence that is the result of known underlying probabilities.

The difference between *haphazard* and *random* in scientific discourse is that the underlying probability base is known or is "knowable" in things characterized as random, whereas it is not in things characterized as haphazard.

Without details supporting the use of "random," it is anybody's guess as to whether the use is justified. Hence, as a reader of results from trials, one should assume *random* means *haphazard* unless the authors provide details elevating the word to the scientific version of random.

A mystical belief exists regarding randomization in trials. It is often seen as "working" if the treatment groups are comparable, and not if they are not. But randomization in trials is not done to yield comparable groups, although on average (across trials), it does a good job of doing so.

Randomization is done to remove selection bias in the assignment process, using a system in which assignments are immune to the wishes or desires of patients and study personnel alike. In the context of trials, the potential for *selection bias* arises when treatment assignments are known in advance of issue and when that information is used to decide whether to proceed with enrollment.

In reference to the treatment groups, we must ask ourselves: Comparable with regard to what? Dozens of baseline characteristics are typically recorded on entry; for a trial participant to be comparable with respect to all such measures is a tall requirement for the equivalent of coin flipping in making treatment assignments.

It is said that God does not throw dice, and so it should be with trialists who want comparability. Randomization is not your ticket if that is what you want. The "solution" (e.g., in a trial involving just one test and a control treatment) is to line up pairs of patients matched on everything you want to be the same and then randomize the members of each pair—one member to the test treatment and the other member to the control treatment—by flipping a coin or its equivalent.

Suppose you want comparability on gender and age. In that case, if you find a male, aged 32, eligible for study, you have to find another one, aged 32, and then randomize the members of the pair.

The downside is that it is tough enough to find patients, one at a time, let alone now in pairs. In short, the approach is impractical because of the added cost and time required for enrollment, to say nothing of the potential difficulty of finding a pair if one is looking for a difficult match (e.g., say, another female, in a predominantly male disease).

Stratification in trials is an active process that goes on during enrollment to classify people into subgroups defined by the variable or variables used for stratification. The purpose is to provide treatment groups that have the same composition for the stratification variable(s).

Say, for example, that you want comparability on gender; that is to say, you want the ratio of males to females to be the same across treatment groups. To accomplish this, you would produce two randomization schedules; one for males and another for females, both with the same assignment ratio. The stratification ensures that the male-to-female ratio is the same for both treatment groups. (Note: Do not confuse equality of the male-to-female ratio across treatment groups with equal numbers of males and females in the treatment groups [see Chapter 8 for a discussion of recruitment quotas].)

Clearly, there is a limit to this kind of imposed balance. It works OK with one or two variables, but its utility as a means of variance control diminishes with the number of variables used and ultimately degenerates to being the equivalent of randomization without any stratification. In any case, the amount of control achieved by stratifying to remove variation is marginal. Stratifying serves no purpose if the variables chosen for stratificaion are not associated with the outcome of interest (often the case).

In my own department, some years back, the introductory course for epidemiology contained an exercise on clinical trials. One of the assignments was for students to look at the distribution of baseline characteristics by treatment group and then to say whether "randomization worked."

Randomization works if the "recipe" for randomization is followed. Indeed, one might examine the distribution of baseline characteristics by treatment group to assess "baseline comparability," but the size of the differences observed alone does not allow one to decide whether a breakdown occurred in the randomization process, any more than getting 70 heads and 30 tails in 100 coin flips would allow you to conclude that the coin was "biased."

The check on whether the recipe was followed is whether assignments were issued as generated by the randomization scheme, and to do that checking, you need an audit trail.

Statisticians like to help randomization along by restricting it. With simple (i.e., complete) randomization, the trialist can end up a long way from the desired assignment ratio when enrollment is finished. For example, consider a trial with a design calling for a one-to-one assignment ratio of test to control assignments. Under simple randomization, one would simply flip a coin every time a person is enrolled.

On average, that system will produce trials with the desired assignment ratio (assuming unbiased coins). But the fact remains that in any particular trial one could, by chance, be far from the desired ratio; for example, 70 people assigned to T (test treatment) and 30 to C (control treatment) in a trial involving 100 people. Further, even if by chance you ended up with exactly 50:50, it could turn out, by chance alone, that most of the flips early on were to T and then later mostly to C, in effect, exposing the results to a time trend if people recruited early on are different from those recruited later on.

The "fix" uses *blocking* to force the assignments to meet the specified assignment ratio at intervals over the enrollment process. For example, suppose you want things to balance after every eight assignments in a trial with a 1:1 assignment ratio. In that case, the ratio would be exactly 1:1 after the eighth assignment, the sixteenth, twenty-fourth, etc., in blocks of the size of eight.

So, suppose in the second block of eight, the assignments for the first six people enrolled was $CCTCTC$. In this case, the coin flipping would stop and the last two people in the block would be assigned to T, so that when filled, there would be exactly four Ts and four Cs. Then, coin flipping would start anew with enrollment of the seventeenth person.

Placebo and Sham Treatments

Placebo is another term subject to confusion and a fair amount of misuse. "Placebo" is the first word in the Roman Catholic office or service of vespers for the dead: *placebo Domino in Regione vivorum* (Psalm 114:9; Vulgate version of the Bible) "I shall please the Lord in the land of the living."

Specifically, *placebo* refers to a pharmacologically inactive substance given as a substitute for an active substance, assuming the person receiving it does not know whether it is active or inactive.

Placebo is used in contexts implying the absence of treatment, but that is generally wrong, to the extent that there is more to treatment than merely administering some substances. Indeed, virtually all trials involving sick people require care. The care, to pass institutional review board (IRB) muster, has to be standard or better. Trials in which care is substandard will not get IRB approval. (See Chapter 9 for description of IRBs.)

Hence, in treatment trials, placebos are overlaid on the usual care provided to all study participants, regardless of treatment assignment.

Placebos come into play in trials in which it is possible to administer treatments in masked or blinded fashion; that is, in which persons do not know if they are receiving an active or inactive substance.

Shams and placebos are first cousins. They are both forms of deception and work as such, but only so long as the person to whom they are administered does not know whether they are real or fake.

Technically, placebos and shams represent "tricks" that delude and, hence, may be used interchangeably. However, for the most part, placebo is used in reference to something taken or applied, as with a pill, liquid, or ointment, whereas sham is usually in reference to some procedure or device, such as the simulation of a surgical procedure.

The importance of a control treatment as a means of identifying a *placebo effect* was recognized by Haygarth (1740–1827) in his 1799 study of Perkins' Tractors, a type of metallic rods.[57] The rods were widely used at the time for a variety of conditions, including crippling rheumatism, pain in the joints, wounds, gout, pleurisy, and inflammatory tumors, as well as for "sedating violent cases of insanity." Haygarth used imitation tractors made of wood on five patients affected with chronic rheumatism.

> Let their [the Tractors'] merit be impartially investigated, in order to support their fame, if it be well founded, or to correct the public opinion, if merely formed upon delusion. Such a trial may be accomplished in the most satisfactory manner, and ought to be performed without any prejudice. Prepare a pair of false, exactly to resemble the true Tractors. Let the secret be kept inviolable, not only from the patient, but every other person. Let the efficacy

of both be impartially tried; beginning always with the false Tractors. The cases should be accurately stated, and the reports of the effects produced by the true and false Tractors be fully given, in the words of the patients. . . .

On the 7th of January, 1799, the wooden Tractors were employed. All the five patients, except one, assured us that their pain was relieved. . . .

The following day Haygarth used the metallic tractors on the same patients.

All the patients were in some measure, but not more relieved by the second application, except one, who received no benefit from the former operation, and who was not a proper subject for the experiment, having no existing pain, but only stiffness of her ankle*.[57]

Data Analysis

Baseline, as an adjective, is concerned with that which occurs just prior to or in conjunction with some event. In the case of randomized trials, the act is randomization for assignment to treatment. Strictly speaking therefore, *baseline data* are data collected on persons in relation to enrollment at or in a period of time prior to randomization—but buyer beware. The reason for the warning has to do with the tendency of trialists to "stretch" the period beyond enrollment, thus opening data to the effects of treatment and, hence, no longer providing a suitable baseline for assessing change.

The *analysis principles* in trials are that the primary analysis should be by original treatment assignment; should include all persons randomized, regardless of compliance to treatment; and should include all events observed, regardless of treatment compliance at the time of the event. The

---

* The tractors were a nostrum developed and promoted by Elisha Perkins (1741–1799); patented in 1796. The tractors were metal rods about 3" in length with a pointed end, made of steel and brass. They were affixed to points of aches or strains on a person's body for "relief". They were widely seen as being useful in relieving a host of aches and pains and were promoted after Perkins' death by his son, Benjamin, in the UK. They remained popular into the early 1800s; used by many, purportedly, even George Washington. For more see http:// www.jameslindlibrary.org/trial_records/19th_Century/haygarth/haygarth_tractors.html)

principles together are often referred to as *intention to treat* (ITT) *analysis*. The trick in reading reports of trials is in trying to determine if this principle was followed.

Readers have to be attuned to language hinting at the fact that the principle was not followed or that investigators are not, as it were, "playing with a full deck." The phrase *per protocol analysis* (PPA) is one such hint. The term is basically a way of noting that the analysis is *not* an ITT analysis. Per protocol analyses are those that ignore the randomization by sorting people by the treatment received rather than the one assigned.

Another word indicating the deck may be short some cards is *evaluable*: for example, as in a paper where the authors restrict the analysis to "evaluable patients." The term should leave one wondering about the results for the "nonevaluables."

Other Commonly Used Terms

- *Off-treatment, off-study,* and *treatment failure* are also words that likely indicate that the investigators have excluded people from analyses. All three phrases basically refer to persons no longer receiving the assigned treatment.
- *Dropout*, in the context of a trial, has two possible meanings: One is that the person has stopped coming to the clinic for visits; the other is that the person was "dropped" from the study because he or she could not, or would not, continue taking the assigned medication.
- The terms *mask* or *blind*, as adjectives in trials, relate to a procedure in which a person, or class of persons (e.g., patients, treaters, or readers in a trial), is not informed of treatment assignment. The world is split into those who use the term *mask* and those who use the term *blind*. Either one works. The advantage to mask is that it avoids the negative connotations and ambiguities associated with blind. Blind carries a connotation of mindlessness or stupidity in some everyday usages (e.g., *blind luck* or *blind stupidity*).

Obviously, *mask* is preferred in eye trials, where blindness may well be one of the outcomes of interest.

- *Single mask/blind* is a condition in which either those being treated or those applying the treatment (but not both) are masked in regard to treatment. Most uses are in the former sense.

- *Double mask/blind* is a condition in which neither the patient nor clinic personnel caring for the person are informed of treatment assignment.

- *Open*, as in an *open-label trial*, is a euphemism for unmasked (i.e., a trial in which treatments are not masked).

- *Open trial* is a euphemism for a nonrandomized trial; for example, one in which the treating physician or the patient him- or herself selects the treatment to be administered.

- *Concealment*, in regard to treatment assignment in randomized trials, refers to the fact that treatment assignments are not known to clinic personnel in advance of assignment. The practice is important in protecting against the possibility of treatment-related bias in the assignment process.

- *Underrepresented* or *understudied*, as used by critics of trials, are value-laden terms implying that investigators failed to include the "correct" mix of people. But, underrepresented in what sense? In regard to numbers in the general population? In regard to numbers having the disease targeted for treatment? In regard to differentials in morbidity or mortality of the disease of interest? The notion of representation has a host of possible meanings. Hence, it is incumbent on the user to define the sense of use.

- The results of trials are usually characterized as *positive* or *negative*. A positive result is one indicative of a beneficial effect. A negative result is one that fails to confirm a prior hypothesis or finding, a result that is opposite in nature or direction to that postulated or desired, or is in reference to a nil result—a result of no difference.

- *Treatment group* refers to a group of persons assigned to receive a specified treatment, as dictated by randomization. Any trial that is internally comparative will have at least two treatment groups: At least one group receiving a test treatment and at least one group receiving a control treatment. The control treatment may be a sham or placebo treatment or simply standard medical care. The control-assigned group may be referred to as the *comparison group* if the treatment is a standard form of treatment, say a drug normally used to treat the condition of interest.

- *Guinea pig,* in reference to people studied, is an evocative, emotion-laden term intended to suggest needless experimentation, experimentation so poorly done that it has no benefit, or use of persons as objects of experimentation involving undue risk or sacrifice. In the context of trials, it is often used in regard to a subset of persons considered to have been denied adequate treatment or to have been exposed to risk without the prospect of offsetting benefit; often in reference to the subset receiving the control treatment in placebo-controlled trials. Most uses in the context of trials, whether or not intentional, have the effect of impugning the judgment of trial sponsors for having funded it and of IRBs and ethics committees for having approved the trial.

- *Informed consent* is a process by which persons eligible for enrollment into a trial are told what is involved, the potential risk and possible benefits associated with participation, the treatments being studied and their possible side effects, and the way in which treatments will be assigned. Often, the modifier, *informed,* is more an expression of wishful thinking on the part of investigators than of documented fact and, hence, is best reserved for settings in which steps are taken to ensure that consent is truly informed.

- *Early stop* refers to a situation in which a trial or a treatment within a trial is stopped earlier than planned, especially because of data suggesting benefit or harm associated with a study treatment.

- *Off-label* as an adjective means being beyond the uses indicated in the drug label insert.

- A *label insert* is a printed document containing information concerning the indication for usage of a drug and its possible side effects, as well as information on mode of action, method and mode of administration, doses and dosages, period of use, and contraindications for use. The insert is prepared as part of a new drug application (NDA) by the manufacturer or marketing agent of the drug. The information provided is subject to the review and approval of the U.S. Food and Drug Administration (FDA). The drug may not be marketed for the named indication without an *approved label*, so named because the document is affixed to the exterior of the package containing the drug (also *package insert*). The insert, as such, is not normally dispensed with prescriptions, but is available on request and can be found in the *Physicians' Desk Reference* (Thomson Healthcare, Inc., ISBN: 1-56363-660-3; 62nd ed.; 2008). Certain classes of drug products (e.g., oral contraceptives) must be dispensed to users with written warnings and precautions.

- The term *endpoint*, meaning an "outcome" or "outcome event," is best avoided. The term is subject to confusion because it is assumed to have operational implications (i.e., that persons experiencing "endpoints" are no longer followed). But usually, protocols call for follow-up and treatment over a defined period of time, even if after an "outcome" or "outcome event."

- An *interim look* is a review of the results of a trial while it is still under way, especially when performed for the express purpose of determining whether the trial should be stopped or modified.

- The descriptor *prospective*, as in "randomized prospective trial" means forward in time and is redundant. Randomized trials are, by definition, prospective.

- *Collaborative* or *cooperative*, as in "collaborative trial," usually is a descriptor meant to indicate that the trial is *multicenter* (i.e., involving two or more different study sites).

- *Controlled*, as in "randomized controlled trial," is largely redundant, because randomized implies controlled.

- *Clinical*, as a descriptor of "trial," is meant to suggest that the study is focused on some clinical condition and carried out in a clinical setting, but there is no guarantee, since "clinical trial" can refer to a wide class of trials, whether or not done in a clinical setting. Usually, the descriptor "clinical" is dropped in favor of descriptors like *field*, as in "field trial," or *prevention*, as in "prevention trial" when reference is to trials involving healthy people.

- The modifier *prevention* (e.g., as in the "XYZ Prevention Trial") implies that the trial involves test treatments aimed at preventing some condition. *Primary prevention trials* are trials involving healthy people not yet having experienced the condition targeted for prevention. Secondary prevention trials are trials involving people who have a history of the condition of interest, where the aim is to prevent reoccurrences of the condition (e.g., in a trial involving persons who have experienced a myocardial infarction, aimed at preventing subsequent myocardial infarctions).
- *Statistically significant* is a characterization applied to results that yield an appropriately small p-value, typically values of ≤ 0.05.
- *Power* is the probability of rejecting the null hypothesis of no treatment difference when, indeed, it is false. Power comes into play when calculating the required sample size for a trial. The goal is to have a sample size that is large enough to provide a reasonable chance (say, probability of 0.8) of detecting a treatment difference when the trial is finished if one exists.

3

The Recipe for Trials

Trials: 19 parts tedium, 1 part fun

CLM

As with Grandma and her apple strudel, there are as many recipes for apple strudel as there are grandmas and no two are alike, although the basic ingredients are the same. By the same token, there are lots of trials, and although no two are alike, the basic ingredients are the same. There is no apple strudel if Grandma does not have the money she needs to buy the sugar and apples for her recipe. Her money comes from her cookie jar or from earnings. Likewise, there is no trial without money to do it. The money here comes from sponsors—generally, a drug company, foundation, or governmental agency.

Trial Sponsorship

In the context here, a *sponsor*, depending on usage can be:

1. A person or agency that is responsible for funding a trial.
2. A person or agency that plans and carries out a trial.

3. The person or agency named in an investigational new drug application (INDA) or new drug application (NDA); usually a drug company or person at such a company, but not always (as with an INDA submitted by a representative of a research group proposing to carry out a phase III or phase IV drug trial not sponsored by a drug company).

Broadly, two things are needed to undertake a trial: a sponsor willing to fund it, and investigators willing to do it. There is no trial without money, and no trial without people to do it. This reality leads to complex "mating dance" rituals, sometimes taking years to consummate.

Suppose you are hankering to do a particular trial. How would you go about the "dance"?

You could, of course, wait for someone to show up at your door and give you the money, but there is no evidence in nature that birds that do not dance survive.

The approach would be for you to "pitch" the trial to attract a suitor. The pitching involves writing applications for funding that outline what is proposed and submitting these to possible sponsors. If the pitching is to the National Institutes of Health (NIH), it is in the form of investigator-initiated grant applications. Applications consistent with the objectives of the NIH are received and subjected to peer review. If they pass muster (only a few do), they are funded and the dance is consummated—but only for a defined period. If the trial is not finished within the period for which it is funded, a new, less elaborate dance commences, to get additional funding to continue or finish the trial.

The alternate is to wait for the sponsor to do a mating dance for a trial of interest to you. This dance is initiated by the sponsor releasing a request for application (RFA) or request for proposal (RFP). In NIH parlance, funding under RFAs is via grants. Funding under RFPs is via contracts. The main difference between the two modes of funding is in degrees of freedoms for investigator prerogatives; typically, this is greater with RFAs than with RFPs. Applications judged "responsive" and adequate are funded.

The fraction of trials initiated by the two types of dances? Not possible to determine with any degree of accuracy because indexing done by the

National Library of Medicine (NLM) is not amenable to such classification. However, it is likely that there is a healthy mix of the two types across the spectrum of trials, with the fraction of sponsor-initiated trials higher for large-scale, multicenter phase III and IV trials than for single-center, small-scale phase I and II trials. (See also Chapter 7.)

Trial Treatments

All trials involve at least one study "treatment" and are done to assess that treatment's value against some standard in curing, ameliorating, or preventing some disease or adverse health outcome.

They all require people who are eligible and willing to enroll to be studied. They all require the collection of data on those enrolled to ascertain the value of the treatments being tested. They all require analysis of the assembled data to determine the value of the treatment being tested.

And they require publication.

Without those five ingredients there is no trial, in the same way that there is no apple strudel if Grandma does not serve it or if she eats it herself.

The "new treatment" may indeed be new in the sense of having just appeared, but it can also be an old treatment used in a new way or used against a new indication.

In the case of drugs, the U.S. Food and Drug Administration (FDA) requires an IND application for testing, regardless of whether the drug is new or old. For example, investigators doing the Alzheimer's Disease Anti-inflammatory Prevention Trial (ADAPT)[2] needed an IND to test celecoxib (Celebrex), a widely used drug licensed for use in pain-relief, and naproxen sodium (Aleve), an over-the-counter pain relief drug because they were being used for a new indication.

Also, "new" does not mean "first," in that there may be several trials ongoing at the same time or over time aimed at testing an agent for use against new indications. For example, a government register of trials yielded a total of 74 studies involving celecoxib that were open for enrollment or getting ready to open for enrollment, as of July 29, 2008 (http://clinicaltrials.gov).

"Treatment" conjures up images of people who are sick, but the reality is that the people in trials may be healthy, and are being treated in the hope of preventing a bad-actor disease later in life, like Alzheimer disease (AD).

The treatment may be a drug, biologic, or vaccine, a medical device, a type of surgery, radiation, diet, exercise, or almost anything thought to have health benefits. In the context of trials, the word *treatment* is simply a generic label to denote a regimen applied to a person in a trial and *treatment group* is simply the generic name for the group of persons assigned to receive a particular treatment in the trial, whether it be the *test* or the *control* treatment and regardless of whether the control treatment be an active treatment or inactive treatment (e.g., as with a placebo or sham control treatment).

Course of Trial

As with recipes for apple strudel, the time involved from start to finish will vary depending on the trial. The median time from start to finish (if by "start" we mean when the first person is enrolled and "finish" when results are published) is probably somewhere between three and four years. "Probably" because reliable data are hard to come by. But whatever they would show, you need to add another year or so if by "start" you mean when the trial was funded and still another year if by "start" you mean when planning (prior to funding) started.

But medians do not tell the whole story. Some trials can be two to three years in the making and may run a decade or longer from start to finish. For example, it was just short of ten years after enrollment of the first patients into the University Group Diabetes Program (see Chapter 15 for a short précis of the trial) before its first results were published,[125,130] and another eight years before its final results on insulin were published.[123]

The promise of benefit must be present to undertake a trial. Trials are done in the hope of showing benefit, not to prove harm, although a fair number end up producing results "on the wrong side of the street." However, that number is not knowable any more than is the number of times Grandma does not serve her apple strudel because it did not "turn out."

The likelihood of trials coming to publication that do not "turn out" is, for certain, considerably less than for those that do. This tendency is part of what is referred to as *publication bias* (a tendency toward publication of results that support conclusions favoring a particular hypothesis or position); in trials, the tendency is to publish results only when they are positive.

The old saw that "the way to cure a disease is to start a trial" is a reminder of the difficulty in recruiting for trials. It isn't that people with the disease suddenly disappear, but rather that they are excluded from study for a variety of reasons—in the parlance of trials, known as *exclusion criteria*. Although every trial involves selection bias, that bias is largely inconsequential if it is the same across treatment groups being compared, as is likely in randomized trials. Exclusions also serve to explain why many trials fall short of their planned enrollment goal and why they invariably take longer than planned.

Grandma needs apples for her recipe. Her favorite is Harrelson, but only after bitten by frost. She picks her own. She is fussy! And so are trialists when it comes to "picking" people for study—but people don't grow on trees! The trialist has to find them one at a time, and even then they can't be "picked" without their consent.

The trialist, when picking people, is driven by competing forces—the force of *exclusivity* and that of *inclusivity*, not unlike those sea monsters of Greek mythology, Scylla and Charybdis, on opposite sides of the Straits of Messina separating Sicily and Italy.

The force of exclusivity comes from the same instinct as Grandma's in wanting to have the same strain of apple, and all uniformly red and plump. The more alike the people enrolled are, the less variation there is likely to be in the way they respond to treatment and, hence, the easier it will be to find a treatment difference if one exists.

Obviously, the trialist has to exclude people not having the diagnosis of interest. They do not need treatment. Even with the diagnosis of interest, the trialist must exclude people in whom treatment is not indicated for whatever the reason. It is not ethical to randomize such people to treatment.

The randomizing trialist must also exclude people who cannot be safely treated with the study treatments. For example, if the trialist is doing a trial involving a placebo or aspirin as study treatments, the trialist has to exclude persons with allergies to aspirin since they might be assigned to receive that treatment. This list of contraindications grows with the number of treatments being tested, to the extent that every treatment has its own unique list of contraindications. Even the placebo treatment can add to the list of exclusions, depending on what it is made of.

The desire for homogeneity in those studied leads trialists to reduce variation by restricting the age range of persons considered for enrollment, by restricting enrollment to persons of a particular ethnic origin, or by excluding males or females so as to eliminate gender as a source of variation. However, the desire for imposed homogeneity comes at a price, in terms of time and effort needed to achieve the desired sample size and in the generalizability of the findings.

All things considered, the best picking routine for the trialist is to be as widely inclusive as medically proper and safe. For the most part, the possible gain in increased precision of treatment comparisons by restriction of who is enrolled is offset by the added costs for recruitment and limitations on the utility of the results.

Data Gathering and Measurement

In the final analysis, the proof of Grandma's apple strudel is in the tasting. In trials, it is in the data. A trial is not a trial without data to evaluate the treatments. But what data? The tendency is to collect everything. This allows for the opportunity to "shop" for the data that proves what one wants to prove (more on this in Chapter 17). The fix is to require specification of the measure to be used for assessment before the trial starts and to stick with that choice when results are analyzed and reported. That measure is what is typically referred to as the *primary outcome measure*.

The measure may be the occurrence of some event or condition or of change. If the latter, the change is measured from baseline (entry into the trial) to some point during or after treatment. For example, in a trial involving drugs to prevent bone loss, the difference can be in a person's bone density at entry versus some point during or at the finish of treatment.

Alternatively, another measure could be occurrence of a bone fracture but, clearly, such a trial would have to involve more people and run longer than one based on density change because fractures (fortunately) are not commonplace.

Obviously, trials with bone fracture as the outcome measure are of higher clinical relevance than are those designed using some substitute measure, like bone density readings, but they are far less common because of the cost and time it takes to do them.

The clinical relevance attributed to the results of trials is related to the outcome measures used to assess treatments. *Clinical relevance*, roughly, is the degree to which findings translate directly to a clinical condition or event. The closer the measure is to the event or condition, the better in terms of relevance. Clearly, results from a trial with fractures as the outcome will be more relevant in deciding whether a drug that increases bone density really reduces fracture rates.

Results of trials can be published anywhere, but the tried-and-true place is in peer-reviewed, indexed medical journals. The indexing is done by the National Library of Medicine (NLM). It indexes some 5,200+ journals published in the US and 80+ other countries as to type of article and content.

Researchers gravitate to indexed journals to display their wares for the same reason that Grandma goes to the County Fair to have her apple strudel judged. But how do the judges know that Grandma actually made the apple strudel? She so attests on an entry form she signs when presenting her apple strudel to fair officials. The *attestation* that the results being presented are the product of the people presenting them for publication is done by assurances they make to editors when submitting the paper, as discussed in Chapter 6.

Grandma is free to make her apple strudel when she pleases, as she pleases, without anyone looking over her shoulder. Indeed, if there are "back seat bakers," she tells them where to go! The situation is different for trialists. They have *institutional review boards* (IRBs); in other parts of the world institutional ethics committees or like names) to answer to.

Trialists are required to have IRB approvals before they can enroll anybody and to have the protocol approved before they start. Changes along the way, inevitable in most trials, as with Grandma when she discovers she has to improvise because she is short on an essential ingredient, must be reviewed by IRBs before they can be implemented, save for a few exceptions (see Question 7; Chapter 23 for one). For more on IRBs see Chapter 8.

It is said that the hardest thing a trialist does is count. It is easy enough to count 1,2,3, ... The hard part is knowing what to count and where to count someone (see Chapter 12 on how not to count). The "recipe," no matter how elaborate, no matter how well-executed, will not generate "fruitful results for the good of society" (see Chapter 8) if the trialist does not count correctly. The basic counting rules for the hard-nosed trialist are:

1. Person counted as randomized are counted the moment the treatment assignment is known to clinic personnel.
2. All persons randomized are counted to the treatment groups to which assigned, regardless of subsequent course of treatment.
3. All events occurring from the moment of randomization forward are counted.
4. Events are counted to the assigned treatment, regardless of degree of treatment compliance at the time of occurrence of events.

These rules are necessary to satisfy the Holy Grail of trials: That the conclusions stated in the primary manuscript be based on the outcome measure designated as primary when the trial was designed (usually the one on which sample size calculations were based) and that the analysis:

1. Be for the treatment groups represented in the trial, as defined by treatment assignments issued in randomization.
2. Includes all patients assigned to the respective treatment groups.
3. Includes all recorded events, regardless of treatment compliance or status at time of occurrence.

4

The Stages of Trials

Never collect more than ten times the amount of data actually needed.

CLM

It is instructive to break trials into stages, somewhat in the same way that one might characterize the activities of Grandma when making her apple strudel from start to finish.

Stage of a trial is different from *phase of a trial*. Stage is a period within the course of a trial. *Phase* is a facet of activities in a sequence of activities related to developing and testing a treatment for possible use in human beings (see Chapter 1 for definitions of phases).

The sojourn times by stage vary depending on the trial. They can be days, weeks, months, or years; months or years in the case of long-term trials, as seen in Table 4.2 for the Childhood Asthma Management Program (CAMP)[22] and the Alzheimer's Disease Anti-inflammatory Prevention Trial (ADAPT).[1]

The difficulty with any ordered set of activities is that they never stay ordered, hence a constant need for backtracking because of plan changes. In the conduct of trials, there is no assurance that activities marked as finished will not reappear anew later on, as for example in a trial already

Table 4.1 Activity stages of trials

Activity stage	Comment
1. Design/funding	Design and funding activities will proceed together in investigator-initiated trials; design is separated in time from funding process in sponsor-initiated trials; ends with initiation of funding
2. Protocol development	Design activities may continue during protocol-development stage; stage ends with start of randomization
3. Patient recruitment	May extend into subsequent stages; ends with completion of patient recruitment
4. Treatment	Will overlap activities of stages 3 and 5; may also overlap activities of stage 6 in trials involving anniversary close-out designs*; ends with last treatment-administration visit for last person enrolled
5. Follow-up	Likely to overlap activities of stages 3 and 4, and activities of stage 6 in trials involving anniversary close-out designs; ends with last scheduled follow-up visit for last person enrolled
6. Close out	May overlap activities of stages 3–5; ends with last close-out patient visit/contact
7. Termination	Starts on completion of last close-out visit/contact; ends when funding ends
8. Post-trial follow-up	Optional; may not occur, and if it does, it may be months or years after completion of the termination stage

*Designs in which persons enrolled are treated and followed for a specified period of time, say 26 weeks, and then separated from the trials in order as enrolled. The other design is one in which separation occurs at the same time, regardless of when persons were enrolled.

enrolling and treating, in which it is decided that another treatment should be added, causing a new set of activities relating to design and protocol development—as happened with the University Group Diabetes Program (UGDP).[124,125]

But even without backtracking, an overlap of activities occurs, as indicated in the listing above. For example, the activities related to treatment and follow-up start as soon as the first person is enrolled and, hence, overlap those in the recruitment and enrollment stage. Indeed, the activities may overlap almost completely when the period of treatment and follow-up per person is short.

Table 4.2 Sojourn times by stage for Childhood Asthma Management Program (CAMP) and Alzheimer's Disease Anti-inflammatory Prevention Trial (ADAPT)

	Start	Finish	Sojourn time
CAMP			
Funding*	Nov 1990	Oct 1991	12 mos
Design/protocol development	Oct 1991	Nov 1993	2 yrs, 2 mos
Patient enrollment	Nov 1993	Sep 1995	1 yr, 11 mos
Treatment & follow-up	Nov 1993	Jun 1999	5 yrs, 7 mos
Close-out	Mar 1999	Oct 1999	8 mos
Termination	Nov 1999	Jul 2008	8 yrs, 8 mos
ADAPT			
Funding*	Feb 1997	Mar 2000	3 yrs, 1 mo
Design/protocol development	Mar 2000	Mar 2001	1 yr
Patient enrollment	Mar 2001	Dec 2004	3 yrs, 9 mos
Treatment & follow-up	Mar 2001	Dec 2004	3 yrs, 9 mos
Close-out	Dec 2004	Jan 2005	2 mos
Termination	Feb 2005	Jan 2010	5 yrs

*For CAMP, start date taken as release date for RFP leading to creation of CAMP; for ADAPT start date taken as three months before first grant submission to the National Institutes of Health for funding ADAPT.

Also, the order of activities will, to some degree, depend on how the trial is initiated. The activities related to funding and design may go on at the same time in investigator-initiated trials, but will be separated in time in sponsor-initiated trials in which, at least for government-initiated trials, only the broad strokes of design are laid out in the request for application (RFA) or request for proposal (RFP), with details waiting until funding has been initiated (see Chapter 3).

Similarly, the termination stage can come any time, sometimes even before the first person is enrolled if the sponsor decides to abort the study. Termination can come in the normal course of affairs, with the finish of treatment and follow-up, or during treatment and follow-up if it is judged to be futile to continue* or that a treatment being evaluated may be harmful.

In reality, the stages are better seen as two-dimensional arrays with activities, as listed below, overlaid on stages, since they run across stages:

- Training and certification
- Data collection and processing
- Monitoring
- Data analysis
- Paper writing

For example, the activities related to training and certification of study personnel for the various activities involved in enrollment, treatment, follow-up, and data collection continue in some form or another to the end of data collection.

Similarly, monitoring for performance in enrollment, follow-up, and data collection starts as soon as enrollment gets under way and continues to the end of the trial. Monitoring for treatment effects starts soon after the first persons are treated and continues until treatment is finished.

Data collection and processing should proceed in lock-step fashion with data generation. That means data have to be keyed when collected, or in short order thereafter, and harvested at regular intervals over the course of the trial for use in performance and treatment effects monitoring and for analyses in relation to paper-writing activities.

Paper-writing in trials is traditionally thought of as an activity that starts after data collection is finished, but that is a misconception, at least in long-term trials. For example, the Coronary Drug Project (CDP) research group produced nine papers before the final results were published in 1975[29] and more than 20 after that. The UGDP produced eight major papers before the final results for the insulin treatments were published in 1978.[122]

Tools for managing and orchestrating activities are checklists, timetables, Gantt charts, and critical path analyses. A *Gantt chart* (after Henry Laurence

---

* Typically, such judgments are based on "futility analyses" in which the focus is on assessing the likelihood that the trial will produce positive results if continued to its appointed end.

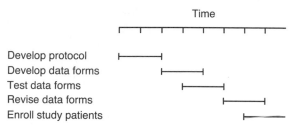

Figure 4.1 Gantt Chart.

Gantt, 1861–1919, American engineer) is a type of graphic display showing activities in relation to time, as illustrated in Figure 4.1. They are especially useful in displaying overlap of activities.

A *critical path analysis* is an analysis of a collection of activities to identify critical elements in that set of activities; it is useful in providing insights as to the order of execution of a complex set of activities in order to assure a timely completion of the entire set. Basically, the critical elements in the conduct of trials after funding are:

- Institutional review board (IRB) approvals
- U.S. Food and Drug Administration approval or acquiescence (if trial requires an investigational new drug application)
- Approval of the study protocol and consent documents by IRBs and study-governing bodies
- Consummated drug supply agreements
- Approved drug packaging, labeling, and distribution schemes
- Tested data collection forms
- Approved patient screening and enrollment procedures
- Tested randomization system

These elements are critical because they affect downstream activities. For example, failure to have IRB approval will preclude any screening for enrollment into the trial. Similarly, in cases in which drug treatments are involved, enrollment is precluded prior to drug availability and being labeled and distributed to clinics for use.

5

The Anatomy of Trials

The whole is more than the sum of its parts.

Aristotle

Required Documents

- Study protocol
- Consent forms
- Institutional review board (IRB) approvals
- Investigator's brochure (in the case of drug trials done under an investigational new drug [IND] application)
- Manual of operations/handbooks
- Data forms/case report forms (CFRs)

Every trial requires a *protocol*. The word is of Greek origin (*prōtokollon*), meaning first sheet of a papyrus roll bearing the date of manufacture and "to hold together" (*prōt-* + *kollon*).

A protocol is a document specifying the eligibility requirements for enrollment, the treatments being tested, the method of assigning people to treatment, and details regarding follow-up and data collection. It is the blueprint for the trial.

The *consent form* is used to document the fact of consent. Ideally, it is written at an eighth- or ninth-grade reading level (easier said than done, especially with the 25-cent words used in medicine) and provides an explanation of the trial, the rationale for doing it, the treatments being tested, what it means to be "randomized to treatment," the potential risks and benefits from being studied, and a statement that persons enrolled are free to withdraw from the trial at any time after enrollment without adverse consequences. (See Chapter 20 for more details regarding consent from the perspective of persons shopping for trials.)

Consent forms are subject to *IRB approval*. To be official, these forms must bear evidence of having been approved and they must indicate the date through which the approval is valid.

For consents to be truly informed, study candidates need to have ample time to consider their decision. It is not in anyone's interest to rush the decision-making process. There is no good achieved if a person enrolls and then drops out because he or she was inadequately informed about the study design or discovers things about the study not made clear at enrollment.

The file of IRB approvals and correspondence is akin to a driver's license. You had better have yours with you if you are stopped by a trooper. Likewise, you had better have an up-to-date IRB file if auditors come calling.

The *investigator's brochure* is provided by the drug company whose product is being tested. It contains information regarding the chemical nature of the drug, its mode of action, and a summary of available animal and clinical data relating to the safety and efficacy of the drug. The manufacturer is obligated to revise and update the brochure as information accrues as to the safety and efficacy of the drug.

The *manual of operations* (MoO) and *study handbooks* are akin to those black notebooks you see pilots looking at before take-off. They contain instructional material for operation of the trial in regard to treatment administration and data collection.

The difference between manuals and handbooks has to do with organization and format. The typical manual of operations is comprised of chapters and is heavy on narrative text. The typical handbook is organized by topic, is light on narrative text and heavy on lists, tables, and figures.

Of the two formats, the handbook format is more user-friendly and easier to maintain and update. It is much more daunting to revise chapters than pages in handbooks (and hence easily put aside).

The *data forms* are the heart and soul of any trial. A one-to-one correspondence must exist between that which is recorded during the data collection process and that which gets keyed into the study data system. Discrepancies have to be resolved.

Funding

Trials are funded by foundations, manufacturers of drugs, biologics, or devices, and by governments. Some clue as to the proportion funded by each can be gleaned from indexing done by the National Library of Medicine (NLM). The NLM started indexing publications by source of funding in 2005. Publication types included:

- Research support, non-US gov't
- Research support, US gov't, non-PHS
- Research support, US gov't, PHS (includes National Institutes of Health [NIH] support)

The ratio of 2009 trials (English-language publications) indexed as involving U.S. government funds to non-US gov't funds is about 1:3 (5,119/15,687 for the publication type "clinical trial," 2,773/8,716 for the publication type "randomized controlled trial," and 606/2,220 for the publication type "multicenter study" and the type "randomized controlled trial"; counts as of October 14, 2010). One can reasonably surmise that the majority of trials not indexed as involving U.S. government funding are industry-funded, but the indexing done by the NLM does not allow for more specific classifications.

Initiation

Funding does not reveal much, if anything, about who initiates trials. In truth, initiation is hard to track. Reports of trials do not usually contain information as to how they came about. There is no indexing in the PubMed system that allows one to track "initiator roles." The output of published trials is a mixture of investigator-initiated and sponsor-initiated trials, but the mixture is unknown. What is certain is that the ratio of investigator-initiated to sponsor-initiated trials decreases as trials progress from phase I to IV and from single-center to multicenter trials.

Consider the way NIH trials are initiated. If investigators are trying to do the initiating, they do that by submitting a grant application to the NIH. Whether the application is funded depends on how it fares against all other applications received by the NIH within a designated time period. If an application receives a fundable priority score (relative to all other applications received and reviewed), it gets funded. If approved, but without a sufficiently high priority score, or if "disapproved," investigators have the option of trying again. If the second attempt does not succeed, they give up (they only get two tries), or they look elsewhere for funding.

If the initiative comes from the NIH, it starts with the release of a request for applications (RFA) or request for proposals (RFP). As noted in Chapter 3, the main difference between the two modes of initiation is in how funding is supplied to investigators—grants in the case of RFAs and contracts in the case of RFPs.

The competition now is for funding from a pot of money earmarked by the institute. Unless the institute ultimately decides to withdraw the RFA or RFP (rare), investigators know that the trial will proceed. The only unknown is whether a particular application will be funded.

Single-center vs. Multicenter Trials

Every trial involves functions related to screening, enrolling, treating, and following study subjects, and to receiving, processing, and analyzing data generated from study subjects. If those two functions go on under the direction of the same scientific head, and the persons performing them are located in the same institution, the trial is a *single-center trial*.

The majority of published trials are single-center trials; about 80% of all randomized controlled trials (12,483 out of 15,604 published in 2007; humans and English publications; counts as of October 30, 2008).

A trial is a *multicenter trial* if the structure for carrying it out involves two or more administratively independent organizational units. This definition is consistent with the one used by the NLM: *work consisting of a controlled study carried out by several collaborating institutions*.

Multicenter trials make up about 20% of randomized controlled trials (3,121 out of the 15,604 in 2007 publications; counts as of October 30, 2008), but what they lack in numbers they make up for in sample size. For example, the median sample size for multicenter randomized trials published in the *Journal of the American Medical Association* (JAMA), the *New England Journal of Medicine* (NEJM), the *British Medical Journal* (BMJ), and *Lancet* in 2006 (194 trials) was about four times larger than for single-center trials (97 trials): 801 versus 203.

What multicenter trials lack in numbers they also make up for in terms of geographic coverage. Many more clinics are involved in multi-center trials than are represented in the aggregate of single-center trials, even though single-center trials outnumber multicenter trials by 4 to 1.

Indication of this reality can be seen in Table 5.1 for the 194 2006 multicenter trials just mentioned. The median number of clinics per multicenter trial was 28 for the 158 trials where counts of clinics were possible.

Sponsor-investigator Roles

Every trial is the product of a partnership between investigators and sponsor. The role of the sponsor in the partnership ranges from:

- **Nil**—For example, as in some investigator-initiated single-center trials funded via the NIH's Research Project Grant Program (RO1) grants

Table 5.1 Number of clinics represented in 2006 multicenter trials published in JAMA, NEJM, BMJ, and Lancet*

No. of clinics	No. of Multicenter trials
No. not specified	36
1	1
2–4	12
5–10	24
11–20	30
21–40	38
41 +	53
Total	194

*Journal of the American Medical Association, New England Journal of Medicine, British Medical Journal.

- **Intermediate**—As in some investigator-initiated multicenter trials funded via NIH cooperative agreements or in NIH contract-funded trials
- **Dominant**—As in some NIH-sponsored trials initiated via RFPs

Table 5.2 indicates the locus of control for activities/functions by initiator role in the trial. *Inv* entries indicate that control of the designated activity/function rests with study investigators. *Spon* indicates that control of the designated activity/function rests with the sponsor, and *Inv/Spon* indicates that control is shared by investigators and sponsor. A transition of control occurs from investigators to sponsor, with transition from RO1 investigator-initiated trials to NIH-initiated trials.

Table 5.2 Characteristics of National Institutes of Health (NIH)-funded trials

	Investigator-initiated		Sponsor-initiated	
Activity/function	RO1 grant	Coop agree*	RFA	RFP
Study leaders				
PI/Study chair choice	Inv	Inv	Inv/Spon	Spon
Study officers designation	Inv	Inv	Inv	Inv/Spon
Study centers				
Clinic selection	Inv	Inv/Spon	Inv/Spon	Spon
Coordinating center selection	Inv	Inv	Spon	Spon
Study protocol				
Eligibility criteria specification	Inv	Inv	Inv	Inv/Spon
Choice of study treatments	Inv	Inv	Inv/Spon	Spon
Data collection requirements	Inv	Inv	Inv/Spon	Inv/Spon
Final study protocol	Inv	Inv/Spon	Inv/Spon	Spon
Governance				
Steering committee (SC) composition	Inv	Inv	Inv	Inv/Spon
Ancillary study policy	Inv	Inv	Inv	Inv/Spon
Publication policy	Inv	Inv	Inv	Inv/Spon
Authorship policy	Inv	Inv	Inv	Inv/Spon
Data monitoring committee				
Appointing authority	Inv	Inv/Spon	Inv/Spon	Spon
Reporting route	Inv	Inv	Inv/Spon	Spon

*Coop agreement = Cooperative agreement: An agreement between an institute of the NIH and a set of investigators that provides a structure for sponsor–investigator cooperation in the design and execution of the trial; funding via U01 or U10 grants.

Organization / governance

Every trial has a scientific head—typiced to as the *principal investigator*[*] (PI) in the case of single-center trials and *study chair* in multicenter trials. Investigator-initiated proposals typically arrive at the NIH complete with study PI or chair designated, with the basic elements of the governance structure specified, and with the line-up of centers for the trial.

The organization/governance structure may be similarly complete in responses to RFAs or RFPs calling for such detail. If such detail is not required in responses, the structure will be fleshed out after centers are funded.

Trials do not run themselves. Without defined and well-oiled organizational and governance structures, they will fail. I have spent years trying to teach aspiring clinical trialists the finer points of governance and organization. But, alas, every time I have tried, I have ended up with more sleepers than Motel 6. Invariably, the nonverbal communication is, "Why are you telling me these things? I am interested in research, not administration!" If I deign to remind them that, as researchers, they can look forward to spending lots of time administrating, I get blank stares. I expect I may be getting the same reaction about now (if you got this far).

The formality and complexity of organizational and governance structures, of necessity, increases as a function of the size and length of trials and as they move from single-center to multicenter. Day-to-day leadership typically rests with persons formally or informally recognized as study leaders; in multicenter trials, these are typically referred to as *study officers* and

---

[*] *Principal* means first, highest, or foremost in rank, importance, or degree; chief. The meaning of the term is murky in contexts referring to multiple persons, e.g., as is sometimes the case in multicenter trials, where the heads of individual centers are referred to as "PIs." Uses where reference is to multiple persons, represents an oxymoron of sorts, but such uses are now commonplace with NIH funding, with the establishment of multiple principal investigator awards for science projects, effective February 2007. (http://grants.nih.gov/grants/guide/notice-files/NOT-OD-07-017.html; NOT-OD-07-017; Release Date: November 20, 2006).

correspond to the study chair, study vice chair (if there is one), director of the coordinating center, and project officer representing the sponsoring agency.

The building block for organizational structures is the committee. Scratch the surface of a multicenter trial and you will find committees, sometimes lots of them. For example, at full maturity, the Coronary Drug Project (CDP) had 14 standing committees.[30]

By the way, this is why *Robert's Rules of Order* makes it onto "A Reading List of a Different Kind" (Chapter 21). It makes the list, not because of a desire to make an aspiring trialist into parliamentarians, but rather to equip the trialist for survival in committee-laden settings. Experience teaches that those schooled in Robert's rules can control discussions and debates by knowing about tabling motions, substitute motions, "call the question," and moves to adjourn.

The key committees in multicenter trials are:

- Steering committee (SC)
- Executive committee (EC)
- Data and safety monitoring committee (DSMC)

The *steering committee* is the premier leadership committee in multicenter trials. It has overall responsibility for conduct of the trial and is the body to which all other committees report. It is typically chaired by the chair of the study, and its membership varies. In trials involving a modest number of centers (say, 12 or fewer), the usual mode of composition is the "one center, one vote" rule, with the heads of the various centers forming the committee. This form of representation becomes unworkable once the number of centers goes much beyond 12. It morphs into a mix of ex-officio positions for study officers and elected members. For example, in the case of the CDP, the center representation model would have eventually led to a steering committee of about 60 people. The actual size was 20, with 17 voting members.[30]

The *executive committee*, when it exists, is variously composed. In some cases, it is synonymous with study officers. In other cases, it may include them and other selected members from the steering committee. It reports to the steering committee, and is primarily responsible for direction of the day-to-day affairs of the study; typically, it is headed by the chair or vice-chair of the steering committee.

The names "steering committee" and "executive committee" are interchangeable where there is just one leadership committee. The body may be referred to as a steering committee in some structures and as an executive committee in others.

The other key committee in most multicenter trials and some single-center trials is the data and *safety monitoring committee* (DSMC), also known as *data and safety monitoring board* (DSMB), *data monitoring committee* (DMC), or *treatment effects monitoring committee* (TEMC). This committee is typically comprised of voting members independent of the trial, and nonvoting members associated with the trial. Members representing the study are typically limited to those from the data center/ coordinating center.

The primary function of the committee is to look at accumulating results from the trial as it proceeds in order to make recommendations for changes, should they be deemed necessary based on accumulating data.

As noted earlier, the relationship of the committee to study investigators becomes more distant as trials progress from investigator-initiated to NIH-initiated.

The issue of who appoints the DSMC and to whom it reports can be contentious. In many senses, the best reporting model is to have the DSMC report simultaneously to the investigators and the sponsor. When the sponsor insists on having the DSMC report to it, it is imperative that there be an ironclad understanding that recommendations will be passed expeditiously from sponsor to investigators, without censorship or alteration.

Other functions of the committee may include performance monitoring and review of the study protocol and amendments prior to implementation.

Meetings

Trials are 20% meetings. A glimpse as to the meeting activities of the Alzheimer's Disease Anti-inflammatory Prevention Trial (ADAPT) can be seen in this list of meetings from 2000 through 2007:

Steering Committee Meetings

Face-to face	14
Conference telephone calls	14
Study officers (mostly via conference telephone)	32
Research group meetings (face-to-face)	14

This count does not include untold numbers of staff meetings at each of the participating sites.

An issue in budgeting for multicenter trials has to do with the amounts requested for travel. Somehow, those travel budgets invariably are seen as an unnecessary "frill" by reviewers, but that view is the product of the maxim that "those who love to travel are the ones who haven't."

The glue that holds a group together is contact, up close and personal. E-mail, conference telephone calls, and video conferences do not substitute for face-to-face contact; contact is essential for training investigators and data collectors, and for maintaining interest and involvement in the trial. There is a tendency to limit travel to study "big shots" but, in reality, the most important people to be in face-to-face contact are those involved in data collection.

6

Authorship and Credits

No author dislikes to be edited as much as he dislikes not to be published.

J. Russell Lynes

The expectation is that Grandma made the apple strudel that she enters in the County Fair. Indeed, the form she has to complete requires her to attest to that fact.

There is a similar attestation process for papers submitted for publication. People named as authors are required to certify that they made substantial contributions to (a) the conception and design, or acquisition of data, or analysis and interpretation of data; (b) the drafting of the article or the critical revision of it for important intellectual content; and (c) the final approval of the version to be published.[65]

All three conditions must be met under the Vancouver Convention requirements for authorship. (The requirements may be found on the website for the International Committee of Medical Journal Editors–ICMJE; www.icmje.org. The convention's name derives from the fact that the first meeting of the group took place in Vancouver, British Columbia, in 1978.[65])

It is a violation of ethics if attestations are false.[33]

Consider the hypothetical Placebo or Serpentine (POS) Trial, a randomized, placebo-controlled, superiority trial designed to answer the question of whether Serpentine is better than placebo for prolonging life in a life-limiting disease in adults. It is a multicenter trial with a sample size of 2,000 (1,000 per treatment group) and with treatment and follow-up for a minimum of five years for everyone enrolled.

The trial has a Project Officer (the individual from the sponsoring agency responsible for dealing with technical, scientific, and administrative issues relating to the trial) and 25 centers:

Centers
    Clinical centers 20
    Resource centers 5
        Coordinating Center
        Central Laboratory
        ECG Reading Center
        DNA and Specimen Repository
        Central Pharmacy
Officers
    Pernelda V. Applebee, M.D. . . . . Study Chair
    Roger W. McFarland, M.D., Ph.D. Study Vice Chair
    Richard L. Harris, Ph.D. Director, Coordinating Center
    Franklin B. Casper, Ph.D. . . . . Project Officer

Among the officers, only Harris heads a center. Applebee and McFarland were appointed by the sponsor and are not associated with any center, and Casper is from the sponsoring agency.

The Steering Committee (chaired by Applebee) consists of 11 voting members:

Elected members serve four-year terms without term limits and with elections every two years, with staggered terms to ensure continuity of elected members.

Study officers 4
    Applebee
    McFarland
    Harris
    Casper
Elected members 7
    Clinic directors   5
    Clinic coordinators   2

Important dates in the development and course of the trial are as listed here:

Request for proposal (RFP) issued for POS Trial . . . . Jun 1999
Centers funded . . . . Jan 2000
Institutional review board (IRB) approval of study protocol . . . . Jun 2000
First person randomized . . . . Feb 2001
Last person randomized . . . . Aug 2003
Last follow-up visit . . . . Jul 2008
Final data set for analysis produced . . . . Oct 2008

As of October 2008, the entire set of personnel involved in the conduct of the trial (the "POS Trial Research Group") numbered 176:

All told, the group, counting departures over the course of the trial, totaled 195 people.

Shortly after compilation of the final data set, Applebee starts work on a manuscript summarizing the results of the trial, but she has a dilemma: Whose work is it? Whose name does she put in the masthead of the paper?

Clinics

Clinic directors 20

Clinic associate directors 20

Clinic coordinators 20

Clinic associate coordinators 20

Other clinic staff 63

Total 148

Resource centers

Directors 5

Associate directors 5

Coordinating center staff 10

Other resource center staff 8

Total 28

Study officers not heading study centers 3

Consultants 2

Total Research Group 176

The issue of names on papers in multicenter trials is always sensitive. Basically, the only way to make people happy is to list their names in the masthead in front of everyone else's. Some of the emotion surrounding authorship can be circumvented by establishing authorship policy early on in the course of the trial, before papers are written. But, alas, partly because of inexperience, the issue of authorship has never been addressed by the POS Trial investigators, so there is no policy to guide Applebee.

She could just list her own name, but that would be politically unwise, not to mention unfair. So, how about listing the four study officers? There is no question that all four of them played key roles in the trial, and having other names listed would give Applebee political coverage. But, if so, in what order? Alphabetic? Reverse alphabetic? Applebee first, then alphabetic?

Applebee first, then negotiated order? Eventually, the order* they arrive at is:

> Pernelda V. Applebee, Richard L. Harris, Roger W. McFarland, and Franklin B. Casper

But there are still political risks because even with four names, the listing is still unfair and not an accurate portrayal of the actual effort involved. An easy "fix" is to add an "and" or "for" to the listing, e.g., as with:

> Pernelda V. Applebee, Richard L. Harris, Roger W. McFarland, and Franklin B. Casper for the POS Trial Research Group

> or

> Pernelda V. Applebee, Richard L. Harris, Roger W. McFarland, and Franklin B. Casper and the POS Trial Research Group

(The primary difference is that with "for," the implication is that the four named people are writing on behalf of the POS Trial Research Group, whereas with "and" the implication is that they are simply members of a larger group.)

The "for" or "and" tag line provides a little political cover for the officers, but not much because being merely listed as part of the POS Trial Research Group is not of much value to those so identified in front of promotion committees.

So, why not list everybody who was anybody in the masthead? Even if the listing is limited to center directors and officers, it still has 27 names,

---

* The reason why order is important is because the first position is most cherished. Promotions committees value that position above all others when evaluating candidates for promotion. The first author is assumed to be the primary author and, hence, usually the one who deals with editors getting the paper published and in answering questions concerning the paper after it is published. The last position, at least in the basic sciences, is reserved for the person heading the "laboratory" in which the work was done. It is important also because people in the 4th position and beyond become "et al." in journal listings; in this case Applebee, Harris, McFarland, et al. The format is imposed by journals to save space in bibliography listings.

with order to be determined. That approach leaves junior people, worried about promotion, out in the cold—some of whom, in truth, had more to do with the work and production of the manuscript than those listed.

So, why list any names at all? Why not just attribute the work to the group that did it—the POS Trial Research Group—without any indication in the paper anywhere who actually wrote the paper?

The advantage is that it avoids "jockeying." Whenever names are listed, whether as authors in the masthead or as members of a writing committee, as indicated in a footnote to the title page or in the credit list at the back of the manuscript, there is competition for a place in the listing. When it comes to one's name, everyone likes to see their names in print except, that is, on the crime or obituary pages.

In a sense, the straight corporate form is the fairest and most accurate form of attribution in multicenter trials. But there is just one problem: Journal editors don't like the form. In fact, the New England Journal of Medicine banned the form in an editorial in November 1991[68], but the ban did not hold. Of the 80 multicenter randomized trials published in the NEJM in 2006, nine had the corporate form of attribution.

A problem editors have with the form is deciding who is qualified to attest to authorship per the Vancouver Convention requirements outlined earlier. The solution sometimes imposed, whether or not a writing committee is listed, is to require attestations and disclosure statements from all center directors, study officers, and members of the steering committee. Another drawback is that the form makes it difficult for promotion committees to judge the individual contributions of persons being considered for promotion.

In theory, the corporate form of attribution allows everyone associated with the trial to list papers from the trial on their respective CVs, but that option is, to a large extent, precluded if a writing committee is listed and the candidate is not a member of the writing committee.

The conventional form of attribution (without the "and" or "for" tag line) was used in 13 of the 80 randomized multicenter trials published in the New England Journal of Medicine in 2006. The modified form with the "for" or "and" tag line was used in 58 of the 80.

The median number of authors listed for the 71 multicenter trials having named authors in mastheads was 13; not much larger than for the

31 single-center trials published in the *Journal* in 2006—10. Thirty-three multicenter trials had masthead listings with 15 or more names; the most was 47 (two papers).

It is a stretch to believe that all 47 people meet the three conditions for authorship as outlined in the Vancouver Convention. Anybody who has ever written a paper knows that 90% of the writing is done by one or two people.

In the end, in the POS Trial, the manuscript was submitted with the "big shot" conventional form of listing with 27 names in the masthead.

But author masthead listings, whatever the format, are only part of the information needed by readers to understand a work. Of even greater importance, especially in multicenter trials, is the credit lists accompanying manuscripts. These lists provide data essential to understanding the results and in regard to how and where the trials were done.

Years ago, I got coaxed into seeing the movie *Who Framed Roger Rabbit?* by my kids. The most interesting part of the film for me was the credits. It has the longest running credits of any film I have seen, and the credits revealed that the film was a technological masterpiece.

In regard to the POS Trial results manuscript, investigators were careful to craft a structured credit list to indicate:

- Officers of the study and their institutional affiliations
- Present and past members of the steering committee and their institutional affiliations
- Voting and nonvoting members of the data monitoring committee and their institutional affiliations
- Names and locations of centers (clinical and resource centers) in the trial, complete with names and degrees of center directors and associated staff and their functions in the trial
- Funding sources and contract numbers

But, sadly, their efforts went largely for naught. The journal editors, to "save space," reduced it to a straight alphabetic listing without any indication of location or role—the operational equivalent of the film makers of *Who Killed Roger Rabbit?* running an alphabetic listing of people involved in the film without any indication of role or function.

High-circulation journals, like the *New England Journal of Medicine*, print credit lists in tiny fonts and often as unstructured, unsorted lists. For example, the paper containing the results of the Digitalis Trial published in the journal in 1997 had a credit list containing 459 names, not even alphabetized.[38]

So, who cares about credits? Readers should, because the information is important when sizing up results from trials, as explained in Chapter 15.

7

The Nature of Trials

Axioms of trials:
Start a trial and the patients disappear.
Start enrollment and the disease disappears.
Publish the results and the trend disappears.

CLM

How many trials are under way right now? How many people do they involve? How many males? How many females? How many elderly? How many children? How many trials will actually come to publication? Of those published, what did they cost?

Interesting questions—but, alas, not answerable. Even if every trial was registered before the start of enrollment, we would still be hard pressed for answers to the questions, no matter what system of registration.

Hence, characterization of the nature of trials has to be based on published trials, as indexed in PubMed.*

---

* The National Library of Medicine, part of the National Institutes of Health, located in Bethesda Maryland, indexes the world's medical literature as published in peer-review medical journals. All told, the PubMed database contains citations to almost 13 million English-language publications published in 1966 through 2007 and an additional 3 million citations for languages other than English.

But relying on published trials for insight into their nature is, in a way, akin to astronomers relying on light from stars to characterize what is in the universe. Obviously, by relying only on light that reaches the Earth, they have no way of knowing how many dead stars there are.

Likewise, trialists looking at published trials have no way of knowing how many were done and not published and, like their fellow astronomers, are forced to rely on information coming to light years after they were born.

An idea of the age of the typical trial when published can be seen by summing the times below (as guess-timated by me).

Estimated times from start to publication of the "typical" trial

Planning to funding	1.00	yr
Start of funding to start of enrollment	0.50	yr
Start of enrollment to finish of data collection	3.00	yr
Finish of data collection to final data set	0.50	yr
From final dataset to production of submission-quality manuscript	0.50	yr
From submission to acceptance	0.75	yr
From acceptance to publication	0.25	yr
From publication to repose in PubMed	0.25	yr
Total estimated elapsed time	**6.75**	**yr**

Table 7.1 gives counts of full-length publications in the PubMed database and the number of such publications indexed to the publication type "clinical trial" (see Chapter 3 for National Library of Medicine definition of the type). The last two columns give the percentages of full-length publications that are clinical trials. The percentages have increased from 2.5% in 1966–1970 to almost 9% in 2001–2005 for English language publications.

Table 7.1 Publication type "clinical trial" (CT) as a percentage of full-length publications*

	All publications		CT publications		% CTs	
Year of publication	English-language	Total	English-language	Total	English-language	Total
1966–1970	277,088	567,111	6,629	9,196	2.4	1.6
1971–1975	367,616	638,355	10,622	14,556	2.9	2.3
1976–1980	467,197	742,255	15,240	20,509	3.3	2.8
1981–1985	609,822	893,695	23,375	28,262	3.8	3.2
1986–1990	792,871	1,101,446	38,651	45,257	4.9	4.1
1991–1995	952,977	1,175,989	66,370	75,831	7.0	6.4
1996–2000	1,172,736	1,374,102	101,990	112,747	8.7	8.2
2001–2005	1,422,402	1,629,031	123,846	132,165	8.7	8.1
2006	346,441	386,165	31,114	32,731	9.0	8.5
2007	366,975	405,177	32,868	34,465	9.0	8.5
Total	6,776,125	8,913,326	450,705	505,719	6.7	5.7

* Excluding abstracts, letters to editors, review articles, and other publication types not containing original results; counts limited to publications tagged by the National Library of Medicine as involving human beings.

Pursuant to the question as to the number of people involved in trials: In 2006, there were 31,114 English-language publications indexed to the publication type "clinical trial" (Table 7.1). If one assumes that the median sample size of those trials was 60, then together they represent results from nearly 2 million study subjects. If one further assumes that for every published trial there are three that are never published, and a median sample size of 30 for those, then the number of study subjects represented is closer to 5 million than 2 million.

Pursuant to the question of the cost represented by the trials published in any given year: Again one can only guess. Suppose the typical trial produces a total of 30 person-years of follow-up data (e.g., as would be the case if one assumes the median follow-up time is 26 weeks and a median sample size of 60). Suppose that the direct cost for generating a person-year of follow-up data (in 2006 dollars) is $15,000, producing a direct cost of $450,000 per trial and a total direct cost of $14 billion for the 31,000 trials. The total cost, including indirect costs, will be considerably higher.

Table 7.2 gives fractions of the publication type "clinical trial" indexed to the publication type "randomized controlled trial" (as defined in Chapter 1), which is around 50% of the publication type "clinical trial" in recent years.

The NLM started indexing "multicenter study" as a publication type in the late 1980s. Table 7.3 gives the percentage of the publication type "randomized controlled trial" indexed to the publication type "multicenter study." The percentage of that combined type represented almost 20% of randomized controlled trials in 2007.

Table 7.2 Randomized controlled trials as percentage of all clinical trials (all languages)

Year of publication	No. CTs	No. Rz CTs	% CTs Rz
1966-70	9,196	1,310	14.2
1971-75	14,555	2,957	20.3
1976-80	20,510	7,594	37.0
1981-85	28,261	13,962	49.4
1986-90	45,256	24,718	54.6
1991-95	75,838	41,200	54.3
1996-00	112,757	51,639	45.8
2001-05	132,366	64,603	48.8
2006	33,532	16,131	48.1
2007	34,101	16,944	49.7
Total	506,372	241,058	47.6

Table 7.3 Multicenter randomized clinical trials as percentage of all randomized trials (all languages)

Year of publication	No. CTs	No. Rz CTs	% CTs Rz
1991-95	41,200	5,606	13.6
1996-00	51,639	8,380	16.2
2001-05	64,604	11,494	17.8
2006	16,131	2,942	18.2
2007	17,138	3,347	19.5
Total	190,712	31,769	16.7

Hints at answers to the question of who pays for the trials can be gleaned from indexing (introduced in 2005) relating to support. As of October 14, 2010, there were 18,155 trials indexed to the publication type "randomized controlled trial," published in 2009 (English language and limited to human trials). Out of those, 2,773 were funded in part or totally by the U.S. Public Health Service (mostly National Institutes of Health funding). The number of reports not listing any U.S. government support was 8,716.

A view reinforced during the women's liberation movement in the 1980s was that women and their diseases were understudied in clinical trials relative to men and their diseases. This concern was sufficient to cause the U.S. Congress (with the NIH Revitalization Act of 1993[94],[95]) to instruct trialists to focus more effort on females. The remaining tables in this chapter relate to the issue of gender representation in trials. (See Chapter 11 for more on gender.)

An indication of gender and age representation in published trials can be seen in Table 7.4 for the publication types "clinical trial" and "randomized controlled trial" for 1990 and 2006 publications. The columns labeled *# male* and *# female* give numbers of trials indexed as involving males and females. The ratios of the two counts are given in the last two columns of the table. Ratios of less than 1.00 indicate more male-only than female-only trials. Ratios of greater than 1.00 indicate the reverse.

Table 7.4 1990 and 2006 publication "clinical trial" (CT) and "randomized controlled trial" (Rz) by age and gender (counts limited to English, human, full-length publications)

	# male		# female		# F / # M	
	CT	Rz	CT	Rz	CT	Rz
1990						
Newborn (birth–1 mo)	99	62	159	106	1.61	1.71
Infant (1–23 mos)	191	112	181	107	0.95	0.96
All infant (0–23 mos)	246	151	295	189	1.20	1.25
Preschool child (2–5 yrs)	314	184	300	177	0.96	0.96
Child (6–12 yrs)	493	277	474	266	0.96	0.96
Adolescent (13–18 yrs)	1,125	704	1,134	732	1.01	1.04
All child (0–18 yrs)	1,420	903	1,468	960	1.03	1.06
Adult (19–44 yrs)	3,931	2,472	3,801	2,439	0.97	0.99
Middle aged (45–64 yrs)	3,599	2,301	3,528	2,252	0.98	0.98
Middle aged (45+ yrs)	3,803	2,438	3,724	2,384	0.98	0.98
Elderly adult (65+ yrs)	2,237	1,408	2,204	1,374	0.99	0.98
Old adult (80+ yrs)	562	343	546	323	0.97	0.94
All adult (19+ yrs)	5,173	3,274	4,989	3,219	0.96	0.98
2006						
Newborn (birth–1 mo)	464	174	637	278	1.37	1.60
Infant (1–23 mos)	970	366	995	381	1.03	1.04
All infant (0–23 mos)	1,179	468	1,356	570	1.15	1.22
Preschool child (2–5 yrs)	1,544	577	1,541	577	1.00	1.00
Child (6–12 yrs)	2,545	1,007	2,559	1,018	1.01	1.01
Adolescent (13–18)	4,736	2,151	4,956	2,256	1.05	1.05
All child (0–18 yrs)	6,151	2,908	6,521	3,106	1.06	1.07
Adult (19–44 yrs)	14,220	6,653	15,140	7,041	1.06	1.06
Middle aged (45–64 yrs)	14,667	6,838	15,365	7,189	1.05	1.05
Middle aged (45+ yrs)	15,917	7,434	16,616	7,802	1.04	1.05
Elderly adult (65+ yrs)	10,346	4,550	10,690	4,694	1.03	1.03
Old adult (80+ yrs)	3,448	1,323	3,502	1,334	1.02	1.01
All adult (19+ yrs)	20,063	9,642	21,069	10,180	1.05	1.06

Indirect evidence of the impact of the NIH Revitalization Act of 1993 on the gender composition of trials can be seen by comparing ratios for 1990 publications with those for 2006. The female-to-male ratios for 1990 publications range between 0.94 and 1.06 for children and adults, and from 0.95 to 1.71 for infants. The corresponding ranges for 2006 publications are 1.00 to 1.07 and 1.03 to 1.60, respectively.

The counts in Tables 7.5 and 7.6 are generated using algebra to classify trials by gender; this was done by identifying trials indexed in PubMed as involving males but not females, females but not males, males and females, and gender unknown.

Table 7.5 gives the gender mix for trials over time. The ratio of female-only to male-only trials has increased for all three types of trials cataloged; for example, from 0.81 in 1966–1970 to 1.56 in 2001–2005 for randomized controlled trials. The pattern is especially striking for randomized multi-center trials, with the ratio standing at 3.13 for 2001–2005 publications, thus indicating a marked female–male composition differential.

There is no reliable way of knowing the actual numbers of males and females represented in trials without hand counting them, since indexing in PubMed does not include information on sample size. However, an educated guess is that the numbers will mirror the ratios of female-only to male-only trials. Hence, if 2 million people are represented in the trials, as estimated above, the female-only to male-only ratio of counts of 1.58 translates to an estimate of 1.16 million females and 0.84 million males studied. In reality, the estimated number of females may be low, given the striking excess of female-only randomized multicenter trials in 2006 (3.44) since multicenter trials involve larger numbers of people than are represented in single-center trials.

The impetus that propelled the U.S. Congress to instruct the NIH to ensure inclusion of more women was due, in part, to the belief that most drugs were developed with predominately white male study populations. Table 7.6 addresses the issue of gender representation in trials as indexed by phase by the NLM (see Chapter 1 for definitions).

As seen from Table 7.6, the majority of trials indexed to a phase involve both males and females. The ratio of female-only to male-only trials is consistently 1.0 or higher, except for phase I and II trials in 1993–1995 for the

Table 7.5 Trials by gender (English language)

Year published	No. trials	M-only	F-only	M&F	Not stated	F-only/ M-only
A. Clinical trials						
1966-70	6,629	14.8	10.8	35.8	38.7	0.73
1971-75	10,622	13.6	9.7	43.4	33.3	0.71
1976-80	15,240	12.3	11.3	48.1	28.3	0.92
1981-85	23,375	11.9	10.8	50.4	26.9	0.91
1986-90	38,651	12.8	11.1	49.0	27.1	0.87
1991-95	66,370	11.5	11.6	58.4	18.6	1.01
1996-00	101,990	10.0	11.5	63.3	15.1	1.15
2001-05	123,846	8.5	11.6	67.2	12.8	1.37
2006	31,114	7.4	11.7	68.9	12.0	1.58
2007	32,867	7.4	11.9	69.3	11.5	1.61
Total	450,704	10.0	11.5	61.2	17.4	1.15
B. Randomized controlled trials						
1966-70	1,122	14.0	11.3	41.1	33.6	0.81
1971-75	2,452	12.3	10.9	47.5	29.2	0.89
1976-80	6,542	13.2	12.0	51.1	23.7	0.91
1981-85	12,374	12.4	11.1	55.4	21.1	0.89
1986-90	21,969	12.7	12.2	53.3	21.8	0.96
1991-95	37,610	12.2	11.6	59.5	16.8	0.95
1996-00	48,292	9.9	12.2	63.4	14.5	1.22
2001-05	61,289	8.3	12.9	66.3	12.5	1.56
2006	15,124	7.7	12.8	68.1	11.4	1.65
2007	16,513	8.2	12.5	68.6	10.7	1.54
Total	223,287	10.1	12.3	62.2	15.4	1.21
C. Multicenter randomized controlled trials						
1986-90	1,128	5.5	9.4	62.4	22.7	1.71
1991-95	5,178	5.1	8.7	70.3	15.9	1.69
1996-00	7,966	4.1	10.4	72.6	12.9	2.52
2001-05	11,131	3.8	12.0	73.0	11.2	3.13
2006	2,895	3.6	12.2	74.5	9.7	3.44
2007	3,263	3.9	11.8	74.8	9.5	3.04
Total	31,561	4.2	11.0	72.4	12.5	2.63

Table 7.6 Gender mix in trials indexed to phase of trial

Year published	No. trials	M-only	F-only	M&F	Not stated	F-only/ M-only
Part 1: Phase I and II trials						
A. "clinical trial" [pt]						
1993-95	3,062	8.3	13.6	63.7	14.4	1.6
1996-00	6,024	7.3	15.0	63.1	14.5	2.1
2001-05	7,769	7.2	13.3	70.2	9.3	1.8
2006	2,041	7.9	14.0	69.9	8.3	1.8
2007	1,718	7.8	10.9	73.6	7.7	1.4
Total	20,614	7.5	13.7	67.4	11.3	1.8
B. "randomized controlled trial" [pt]						
1993-95	459	12.0	6.8	64.9	15.3	0.6
1996-00	1,023	9.2	11.3	62.3	17.2	1.2
2001-05	1,357	9.8	9.8	68.8	11.6	1.0
2006	452	10.4	10.4	67.5	11.7	1.0
2007	481	10.6	7.9	70.5	11.0	0.7
Total	3,772	10.1	9.7	66.6	13.5	1.0
C. "multicenter study" [pt] AND "randomized controlled trial" [pt]						
1993-95	132	3.0	6.8	73.5	16.7	2.3
1996-00	318	4.4	11.3	70.8	13.5	2.6
2001-05	529	4.7	14.2	69.0	12.1	3.0
2006	164	3.7	11.6	75.6	9.1	3.2
2007	189	6.3	5.8	78.8	9.0	0.9
Total	1,332	4.6	11.3	72.1	12.1	2.5
Part 2: Phase III and IV trials						
A. "clinical trial" [pt]						
1993-95	414	6.5	11.6	63.8	18.1	1.8
1996-00	997	8.2	14.3	59.8	17.7	1.7
2001-05	1,673	6.4	17.4	63.7	12.5	2.7
2006	477	3.6	22.4	65.0	9.0	6.3
2007	583	5.3	17.7	65.5	9.8	3.3
Total	4,144	6.4	16.7	63.2	13.5	2.6

(continued)

Table 7.6 Gender mix in trials indexed to phase of trial (cont'd)

Year published	No. trials	M-only	F-only	M&F	Not stated	F-only/ M-only
B. "randomized controlled trial" [pt]						
1993-95	287	8.4	12.5	61.7	17.4	1.5
1996-00	739	7.3	16.0	60.1	16.6	2.2
2001-05	1,301	6.5	19.2	63.0	11.4	3.0
2006	388	3.4	25.3	63.7	7.7	7.5
2007	486	5.8	19.1	65.6	9.5	3.3
Total	3,201	6.3	18.6	62.7	12.4	2.9
C. "multicenter study" [pt] AND "randomized controlled trial" [pt]						
1993-95	142	9.9	11.3	65.5	13.4	1.1
1996-00	417	5.3	16.5	64.5	13.7	3.1
2001-05	805	5.5	22.0	63.2	9.6	4.0
2006	240	2.1	25.4	66.7	5.8	12.2
2007	293	3.8	16.7	72.0	7.5	4.5
Total	1,897	5.1	19.6	65.5	9.2	3.9

type "randomized controlled trial." Some ratios are 3.0 or higher, with the largest ratios appearing for multicenter randomized controlled trials.

Table 7.7 gives the percentage of all NIH dollars spent on predominately women's diseases and conditions versus men's diseases and their conditions. The ratio of female-to-male expenditures has been 1.70 or higher over the time such data have been tracked.

Table 7.7 National Institutes of Health (NIH) expenditures for gender-specific and gender-related research; % of all NIH expenditures (via Office of Research on Women's Health)

FY	Female	Male	F/M
1988	9.7	4.4	2.20
1989	9.9	4.6	2.15
1990	9.7	4.5	2.16
1991	10.0	5.6	1.79
1992	10.7	6.3	1.70
1993	14.3	6.7	2.13
1994	14.5	6.0	2.42
1995	16.1	6.2	2.60
1996	16.0	5.7	2.81
1997	16.2	6.1	2.66
1998	16.0	6.1	2.62
1999	15.5	6.4	2.42
2000	15.5	6.4	2.42
2001	14.7	7.6	1.93
2002	14.9	7.9	1.89
2003	13.5	5.8	2.33
2004	12.7	5.8	2.19
2005	12.8	5.9	2.17

8

The Ethics of Trials

Primum non nocere.

Origin unknown

The modern-day code for research on human beings, the Nüremberg Code, grew out of the Nüremberg War Crime trials; it was set forth in 1947 and is reproduced below.[72,114] It consists of 495 words and ten items. Subsequent codes, most prominently those produced by the World Medical Association (WMA), have grown in length, but the essence remains the same*:

1. The voluntary consent of the human subject is absolutely essential.

   This means that the person involved should have legal capacity to give consent; should be so situated as to be able to exercise free power of choice, without the intervention of any element

---

* The first code of the WMA was promulgated June 1964, in Helsinki. It has been revised several times since, growing in length from 11 paragraphs and 814 words to 32 paragraphs and slightly more than 2,000 words, with the last revision in 2000. All editions are known as the Declaration of Helsinki, after the place where the first edition was produced.

of force, fraud, deceit, duress, overreaching, or other ulterior form of constraint or coercion; and should have sufficient knowledge and comprehension of the elements of the subject matter involved as to enable him to make an understanding and enlightened decision. This latter element requires that before the acceptance of an affirmative decision by the experimental subject there should be made known to him the nature, duration, and purpose of the experiment; the method and means by which it is to be conducted; all inconveniences and hazards reasonably to be expected; and the effects upon his health or person which may possibly come from his participation in the experiment.

The duty and responsibility for ascertaining the quality of the consent rests upon each individual who initiates, directs or engages in the experiment. It is a personal duty and responsibility which may not be delegated to another with impunity.

2. The experiment should be such as to yield fruitful results for the good of society, unprocurable by other methods or means of study, and not random and unnecessary in nature.

3. The experiment should be so designed and based on the results of animal experimentation and a knowledge of the natural history of the disease or other problem under study that the anticipated results will justify the performance of the experiment.

4. The experiment should be so conducted as to avoid all unnecessary physical and mental suffering and injury.

5. No experiment should be conducted where there is an a priori reason to believe that death or disabling injury will occur except, perhaps, in those experiments where the experimental physicians also serve as subjects.

6. The degree of risk to be taken should never exceed that determined by the humanitarian importance of the problem to be solved by the experiment.

7. Proper preparations should be made and adequate facilities provided to protect the experimental subject against even remote possibilities of injury, disability, or death.

8. The experiment should be conducted only by scientifically qualified persons. The highest degree of skill and care should be required through all stages of the experiment of those who conduct or engage in the experiment.

9. During the course of the experiment, the human subject should be at liberty to bring the experiment to an end if he has reached the physical or mental state where continuation of the experiment seems to him to be impossible.

10. During the course of the experiment the scientist in charge must be prepared to terminate the experiment at any stage, if he has probable cause to believe, in the exercise of the good faith, superior skill and careful judgment required of him, that a continuation of the experiment is likely to result in injury, disability, or death to the experimental subject.

The Belmont Report (named after the place where it was drafted; the Belmont Conference Center, Elkridge, Maryland)—the product of the National Commission for the Protection of Human Subjects of Biomedical and Behavioral Research[93]—sets forth basic principles that are to apply when approaching persons for study: these are the principles of beneficence, justice, and respect for persons.[72]

- **beneficence**—A principle in medical ethics that asserts that the options available in treating or caring for one's fellow human being are limited to those justifiable on the basis of the intent to do good.
- **justice**—A principle in medical ethics that asserts that the care and treatment performed or offered in a research setting involving human beings must be done in a just and equitable fashion, not to the benefit of a few or to the exclusion of many.
- **respect for persons**—A principle in medical ethics that asserts that the care and treatment performed or offered to persons in research settings must be done in fashions denoting respect for persons.

The Commission grew out of a firestorm of outrage, brought to the fore in the mid-1960s, from accounts of a few celebrated studies; among them, one involving infecting "mentally defective" children in the Willowbrook State Hospital in New York with hepatitis and another involving the injection of live cancer cells into patients in the Jewish Chronic Disease Hospital in New York City.[72] A publication by Beecher in the *New England Journal of Medicine* in 1966[14] focused attention on the issue of ethics in clinical research.

The outrage led to the Surgeon General of the U.S. Public Health Service to announce, on February 8, 1966, that henceforth National Institutes of Health grantees would have to provide evidence of procedures and practices designed to ensure documented informed consent from persons studied in order to receive funding. The order and implementation of it eventually led to the creation of institutional review boards (IRBs; see Chapter 9 for details on membership requirements for IRBs). Institutional review boards, basically an American creation, exist now around the world, even if by different names (e.g., *ethics review committee* or *Helsinki committee*).

- **institutional review board** (IRB)—A board set forth in regulations emanating from the U.S. Public Health Service for reviewing and approving research involving human beings; the board resides in the institution where appointed; review focuses on the ethics and legitimacy of proposed research from the perspective of risk–benefit for participants and on the adequacy of safeguards for limiting risk; risk may be a direct consequence of procedures performed or may be an indirect consequence of involvement, including risks of invasion of privacy or breaches of confidentiality of persons studied. Technically, the regulations apply only to projects funded by the U.S. government, but most institutions require IRB review of all research involving human beings, regardless of funding source. Also known as *ethics committee, ethics review board, Helsinki committee*.

In the United States, there is no central IRB (unlike in some other regions of the world). That means, in the case of multicenter trials, that there may be as many IRB submissions and reviews as there are centers conducting those trials. The number of submissions can run into the hundreds in some large-scale multicenter trials (e.g., as in a trial of the Digital Investigation Group Trial).[23,38] The closest approximation to a central IRB, in which all centers in a trial clear through the same IRB, is a common IRB, to which all centers in a trial not having their own IRB are shunted to the same free-standing commercial IRB. (See www.circare.prg/info/commerialibr.htm for list.) Investigators at institutions with their own IRBs must use the IRB they are required to use by their own institution.

For trials to clear IRBs, evidence must be presented that the risks and nuisances of being studied are commensurate with the prospects of benefit, and that such prospects outweigh those of harm from being studied. Researchers are barred from doing trials in which those risks outweigh the prospects of benefit.

Investigators and sponsors wishing to mount randomized trials have to be able to argue convincingly that there is a legitimate underlying state of clinical equipoise regarding the treatments to be tested. *Clinical equipoise,* as discussed by Benjamin Freedman,[50] is a state in which knowledgeable people are in a collective state of doubt regarding the proper choice or course of treatment. The state allows for differences of opinion as to proper course, so long as, together, those differences can be seen as a legitimate collective state of doubt.*

The ethical base for randomizing persons to treatment in superiority trials rests on the fact that a legitimate state of doubt exists as to the merits of the treatments being evaluated relative to the comparator treatment. So, for example, if persons diagnosed as having a given disease are to be randomized to receive Treatment T or Treatment C, for randomization to meet ethical muster, investigators must be satisfied that medical opinion is divided as to choice and must be able to satisfy IRBs that this is so.

If the randomization is to Drug T or to a placebo or sham treatment, investigators and IRBs have to be satisfied that no established treatment exists for the disease of interest and that there are legitimate reasons to question the value of Drug T for use against the disease.

---

* The concept of clinical equipoise is a useful construct for dealing with superiority and equivalence trials but is not in rationalizing so-called noninferiority trials, in which the goal is to show that a study treatment is not decidedly inferior to the comparison treatment.

A sustained state of legitimate doubt over the course of a trial, especially in long-term trials, is a theoretical abstraction. Collective states of doubt wax and wane with the ebb and flow of information. That ebb and flow can affect the way clinic personnel proceed in regard to enrolling, treating, and following patients. A "fix" in regard to interim results* from a trial is to shield clinic personnel from such results. Under so-called *blackout modes* of operation, clinic personnel are not privy to interim results. They do not see results until the trial is finished or stopped. The job of monitoring for treatment differences is vested in a body independent of clinics, as discussed in Chapter 5.

This "fix" reduces the risk of people responsible for seeing study subjects in a trial from being influenced by interim results from the trial; obviously, there is no way of shielding them from results reported from other studies during the trial.

Another ethic underlying trials is the *publication ethic*. The second item in the Nüremberg Code states that: "The experiment should be such as to yield fruitful results for the good of society, unprocurable by other methods or means of study, and not random and unnecessary in nature."

One can argue that there are no *fruitful results for the good of society* unless results are published for repose in the libraries and publication databases of the world. People are enrolled in trials with the explicit or implicit promise that, even if they are not benefited from being studied, others may be. That promise is broken when results are not published. The publication ethic obliges investigators to publish, regardless of outcome or direction of results and to do so even for "busted" trials.

In theory, IRBs should not approve studies in the absence of commitments from investigators to publish, but even if they are so required, they would be hard put to enforce the commitment. Further, even if investigators are resolute in that commitment, there is no guarantee that they will find a journal willing to accept their results.

---

* The term *interim result* has various meanings, but in this context refers to reviews of accumulating data from within a trial at various points over its course in order to assess treatment effect; done by comparing treatment groups for outcomes of interest; typically done in relation to treatment effects monitoring, as discussed in Chapter 5 .

There is also an *ethic of recruitment* in trials. That ethic is implicit to the principle of justice, as set forth in the Belmont Report:

Justice is relevant to the selection of subjects of research at two levels: the social and the individual. Individual justice in the selection of subjects would require that researchers exhibit fairness: thus, they should not offer potentially beneficial research only to some patients who are in their favor or select only "undesirable" persons for risky research. Social justice requires that distinction be drawn between classes of subjects that ought, and ought not, to participate in any particular kind of research, based on the ability of members of that class to bear burden and on the appropriateness of placing further burdens on already burdened persons. Thus, it can be considered a matter of social justice that there is an order of preference in the selection of classes of subjects (e.g., adults before children) and that some classes of potential subjects (e.g., the institutionalized mentally infirm or prisoners) may be involved as research subjects, if at all, only on certain conditions.

The report goes on to note that:

Injustice may appear in the selection of subjects, even if individual subjects are selected fairly by investigators and treated fairly in the course of research. Thus injustice arises from social, racial, sexual, and cultural biases institutionalized in society. Thus, even if individual researchers are treating their research subjects fairly, and even if IRBs are taking care to assure that subjects are selected fairly within a particular institution, unjust social patterns may nevertheless appear in the overall distribution of the burdens and benefits of research. Although individual institutions or investigators may not be able to resolve a problem that is pervasive in their social setting, they can consider distributive justice in selecting research subjects.[93]

The *principle of distributive justice* means, among other things, that trialists should forego demographic-based exclusions unless necessary for medical-legal reasons. Indeed, IRBs are to be disposed to challenge demographic-based exclusions and to withhold approvals if such exclusions are not justifiable.

There has been a preoccupation in recent years on gender representation in trials, driven, in large measure, by the belief that women and their diseases have been understudied relative to men. This has led some (e.g., Hayes and Redberg in an editorial in the *Mayo Clinic Proceedings*), to suggest that, "All clinical studies should strive to include equal numbers of female and male participants or to at least reflect the prevalence of the condition of interest by sex."[56]

The trouble with such a standard is that it is open to question on ethical grounds, in that it leads to rejection on the basis of demographics. For example, if the goal is to enroll equal numbers of males and females, the trialist must ultimately exclude on basis of gender when the required number of males or females has been enrolled. The same is true if the goal is to enroll the gender mix as seen in the general population, since that mix may not be the one flowing past the doors of clinics enrolling in the trial.

The standard is predicated on the assumption that trials have to be microcosms of the universe to be a value. Such a requirement would markedly increase the cost of trials and, hence, decrease the number of trials done, assuming static research budgets.

The issue of pay, whether it be to parties for finding persons for enrollment into trials or to persons on or after enrollment, raises troubling ethical issues. The practice of paying finder's fees for referring persons for enrollment has been the subject of a report from the U.S. Department of Health and Human Services Office of Inspector General (2000) entitled *Recruiting Human Subjects: Pressures in Industry-Sponsored Trials* (http://oig.hhs.gov/oei/reports/oei-01-97-00195.pdf). Concerns have to do with the corrosive effect such practices can have on consent processes. The prospect of payment to the study site increases the likelihood of coercive consents. Institutional review boards can be expected to look askance at such practices.

Likewise, pay to persons enrolled, if in more than token amounts, has the potential for causing those persons to accept risks that they would not otherwise accept and causing them to stay in studies from which they would otherwise withdraw. Institutional review boards are sensitive to this issue. They are disposed to making certain that if payment is offered (apart from monies paid to persons to cover expenses incurred getting to and from study sites) it is not large enough to tempt persons to accept risks that they otherwise would not accept.

9

Regulation of Trials

If you have ten thousand regulations, you destroy all respect for the law.

Winston Churchill

Table 9.1 gives a concise chronology of requirements/guidelines pursuant to research on human beings, with emphasis on clinical trials. Some of the important highlights in the regulation of trials include:

- **Documented informed consent**—This requirement became effective with a memo from the U.S. Public Health Service (USPHS) Surgeon General informing recipients of National Institutes of Health (NIH) funding that informed consent would be a condition for funding.
- **Creation of IRBs and review requirements**—U.S. Code of Federal Regulations promulgated the establishment of institutional review boards (IRBs) and review procedures.
- **"Valid" analysis requirement for trials**—*It is the policy of NIH that women and members of minority groups and their subpopulations must be included in all NIH-supported biomedical and behavioral research projects involving human subjects, unless a clear and compelling rationale and justification establishes to the*

Table 9.1 Landmark dates in the regulation of research and trials

Requirement/Guideline	Date
Documented informed consent	1966
Creation of IRBs and review requirements	1974
Valid analysis requirement for trials	1998
Treatment effects monitoring guideline	1998
Adverse event summary reports to monitoring committees	1999
Conflict of interest disclosure	2000
Institutional review board investigator training and certification	circa 2000
Health Insurance Portability and Accountability Act (HIPAA) investigator training	circa 2003
Public data sharing	2003
Registration of trials	2004
Effort reporting	circa 2005
PubMed Central manuscript deposit	2008

satisfaction of the relevant Institute/Center Director that inclusion is inappropriate with respect to the health of the subjects or the purpose of the research. (NIH Guidelines on the Inclusion of Women and Minorities as Subjects in Clinical Research; release date, August 2, 2000; Notice: OD-00–048; updated October 9, 2001; Notice: NOT-OD-02–001)

- **Treatment effects monitoring guidelines**—*It is the policy of the NIH that each Institute and Center (IC) should have a system for the appropriate oversight and monitoring of the conduct of clinical trials to ensure the safety of participants and the validity and integrity of the data for all NIH-supported or conducted clinical trials. The establishment of the data safety monitoring boards (DSMBs) is required for multisite clinical trials involving interventions that entail potential risk to the participants. The data and safety monitoring functions and oversight of such activities are distinct from the requirement for study review and approval by an Institutional Review Board*

(IRB). (http://grants.nih.gov/grants/guide/notice-files/NOT98-084. html)

- Adverse event summary reports to monitoring committees— Effective July 1, [1999]: *all multisite trials with data safety monitoring boards are expected to forward summary reports of adverse events to each IRB involved in the study. This action in no way reduces the responsibilities of individual IRBs to address such reports coming to them from the site over which they have responsibility. NIH program staff will ensure that this language appears in new solicitations for clinical trials and is broadly disseminated to current principal investigators with appropriate follow-up.*
- Conflict of interest disclosure: Institutions receiving PHS funds required to establish and maintain procedures for periodic reporting of conflicts of interest and for determining whether conflicts reported sufficient to disqualify persons from funding.
- Institutional review board investigator training and certification—Required all key study personnel listed on study proposals submitted to IRBs, to demonstrate they understand the ethical principles underlying research involving human beings.
- Health Insurance Portability and Accountability Act (HIPAA) investigator training—: Requirement imposed by universities, colleges, and research institutions to ensure researchers understand and practice those procedures necessary to ensure the privacy and confidentiality of protected health information collected or obtained from study subjects; the requirement was an outgrowth of HIPAA, which was signed into law August 1996.
- Public data sharing—Investigators submitting applications for funding to the NIH after October 1, 2003 were required to include a plan for public data sharing or state why such sharing is not possible; the requirement was limited to requests of $500,000 or more in direct costs in any year of requested support.
- Registration of trials—After July 1, 2005, the International Committee of Medical Journal Editors (ICMJE) required of all trials starting enrollment after that date that: *member journals will require, as a condition of consideration for publication* [of trials], *registration in a public trials registry.*

- **Effort reporting**—Required of persons in universities, colleges, and research institutions receiving U.S. Federal funds for conduct of research; persons are required to certify, under penalty of law if not correct, that effort corresponds to salary allocation.
- **PubMed Central manuscript deposit**—On or after May 2, 2005, investigators producing publications of works funded by NIH were required to submit electronic versions of such publications for deposit in PubMed Central; deposits were to be made within 12 months of publication. (PubMed Central is a free digital database maintained by the National Library of Medicine.)

Regulations and guidelines specific to clinical trials include:

- **Investigational new drug application** (INDA)—Required for any "new drug" (see Chapter 3) being tested for an indication not covered in existing U.S. Food and Drug Administration (FDA) market approvals
- **Data and safety monitoring** (aka, treatment effects monitoring)— Guideline issued in 1998, pertaining to NIH-funded multisite clinical trials involving interventions entailing risk potential to study participants; required directors of NIH institutes and centers to ensure that such trials have monitoring bodies or committees constituted to perform periodic reviews of accumulating data to ensure the safety and well-being of study participants. The requirements of such monitoring were in addition to requirements necessary for reviews and approvals of IRBs.
- **Registration of trials**—Registration of trials in a public registry [34] was put forth as a condition for the publication of results in journals represented by editors of the ICMJE. The regulation applied to trials starting enrollment after July 1, 2005,[132] and could be done in any one of several public registration sites
- **Adverse event reporting**—Effective July 1, 1999, all multisite trials with data safety monitoring bodies were expected to forward summary reports of adverse events to each IRB of record for such trials.

- Consolidated Standards of Reporting Clinical Trials (CONSORT) reporting standard—Adopted by various journals, these standards relate to the contents of published reports of randomized trials.[15,81,87,109]

Institutional Review Boards (IRB)

The IRB is the gatekeeper for human research. Institutional review boards are an outgrowth of the celebrated abuses carried out in the name of human research, and brought to light in the 1960s, as discussed in Chapter 8. The inexorable march to the creation of IRBs started with release of a memo from the Surgeon General of the USPHS (dated February 8, 1966) to recipients of NIH funding notifying them that further funding would be contingent on their being able to provide evidence of procedures and practices having been implemented to ensure the documented and informed consent of all persons studied.[72]

An IRB is a committee or board, emanating from USPHS guidelines and regulations concerning research involving human beings,[72,100] appointed by the administrative authorities of a research institution and constituted to review and approve studies to be carried out on human beings by investigators from that institution. The review focuses on the ethics and legitimacy of the proposed research from the perspective of risk–benefit and adequacy of the proposed safeguards for persons to be studied. The risk may be a direct consequence of study procedures or an indirect one (c.g., as a consequence of the invasion of one's privacy or breach of confidentiality). The review deals with (but is not restricted to) the nature and adequacy of the proposed consent process and related consent statement when there is to be contact with study subjects; in all cases, whether or not such contact occurs, a review of the adequacy of procedures must be done to preserve privacy and confidentiality.

A *human being*, for the purpose of IRB regulations, is a living person about whom an investigator (whether professional or student) conducting research obtains (a) data through intervention or interaction with the individual; or (b) identifiable private information.

Research, for purposes of regulation, is defined as "systematic investigation, including research development, testing and evaluation, designed to develop or contribute to generalizable knowledge." The definition applies regardless of whether or not such "systematic investigation" is ultimately intended for publication and even if done in relation to some demonstration or service program not considered to be research (http://www.hhs.gov/ohrp/humansubjects/guidance/45cfr46.htm#46.102).

Research is considered to "involve" human beings even if the researcher has no contact with the persons being studied. Involvement occurs if the research involves data or records generated on living persons, even if such data or records are available to the researcher without direct contact with persons (e.g., as in a study based on information contained in medical records).

Originally, IRB coverage was limited to research funded by the federal government but now, institutions having federalwide assurances (FWAs) are required to provide IRB coverage of all research meeting the above definitions regardless of funding source and including those not involving any funding.

Federalwide assurance (FWA) is a document filed by an institution engaged in research on human beings; it sets forth methods and procedures to be employed by the institution to protect the rights of study subjects, for minimizing risks of harm for study subjects, and for protecting study subjects from harm. It is applicable to all research conducted by people in the institution regardless of funding sources.

IRB Membership Requirements

The requirements for IRB membership, as set forth in CFR Title 45; Part 46 (revised June 23, 2005) are:

§46.107 IRB membership

(a). Each IRB shall have at least five members, with varying backgrounds to promote complete and adequate review of research activities commonly conducted by the institution. The IRB shall be sufficiently qualified through the experience and expertise of its members, and the diversity of the members, including consideration of race, gender, and cultural backgrounds and sensitivity to such issues as community attitudes, to promote respect for its advice and counsel in safeguarding the rights and welfare of human subjects. In addition to possessing the professional competence necessary to review specific research activities, the IRB shall be able to ascertain the acceptability of proposed research in terms of institutional commitments and regulations, applicable law, and standards of professional conduct and practice. The IRB shall therefore include persons knowledgeable in these areas. If an IRB regularly reviews research that involves a vulnerable category of subjects, such as children, prisoners, pregnant women, or handi-capped or mentally disabled persons, consideration shall be given to the inclusion of one or more individuals who are knowledge-able about and experienced in working with these subjects.

(b). Every nondiscriminatory effort will be made to ensure that no IRB consists entirely of men or entirely of women, including the institution's consideration of qualified persons of both sexes, so long as no selection is made to the IRB on the basis of gender. No IRB may consist entirely of members of one profession.

(c). Each IRB shall include at least one member whose primary concerns are in scientific areas and at least one member whose primary concerns are in nonscientific areas.

(d). Each IRB shall include at least one member who is not otherwise affiliated with the institution and who is not part of the immediate family of a person who is affiliated with the institution.

(e). No IRB may have a member participate in the IRB's initial or continuing review of any project in which the member has a conflict-ing interest, except to provide information requested by the IRB.

(f). An IRB may, in its discretion, invite individuals with competence in special areas to assist in the review of issues which require expertise beyond or in addition to that available on the IRB. These individuals may not vote with the IRB.

(http://www.hhs.gov/ohrp/humansubjects/guidance/45cfr46. htm#46.107)

10

Research Misconduct

*Whoever is detected in a shameful fraud is ever after not believed,
even if they speak the truth.*

Phaedrus

Being able to perform research upon human beings is a privilege born of a public trust. The willingness of societies to grant that privilege is diminished by acts disrespectful of that trust. Any such act, anywhere, serves to erode that trust everywhere. Hence, persons anywhere doing research on human beings have a solemn duty to honor that trust for the good of all.

Research misconduct as defined in 42 CFR Parts 50 and 93 in the Code of Federal Regulations, is:

> Fabrication, falsification, or plagiarism in proposing, performing, or reviewing research, or in reporting research results. (a) Fabrication is making up data or results and recording or reporting them. (b) Falsification is manipulating research materials, equipment, or processes, or changing or omitting data or results such that the research is not accurately represented in the research record. (c) Plagiarism is the appropriation of another person's ideas, processes, results, or words without giving appropriate credit. (d) Research misconduct does not include honest error or differences of opinion.[35]

The Oxford English Dictionary[92] defines fraud as:

1. The quality or disposition of being deceitful; faithlessness, insincerity. 2. Criminal deception; the using of false representations to obtain an unjust advantage or to injure the rights or interests of another. 3. An act or instance of deception, an artifice by which the right or interest of another is injured, a dishonest trick or stratagem. 4. A method or means of defrauding or deceiving; a fraudulent contrivance; in modern colloquial use, a spurious or deceptive thing.

Black's Law Dictionary[17] defines fraud as:

An intentional perversion of truth for the purpose of inducing another in reliance upon it to part with some valuable thing belonging to him or to surrender a legal right. A false representation of a matter of fact, whether by words or by conduct, by false or misleading allegations, or by concealment of that which should have been disclosed, which deceives and is intended to deceive another so that he shall act upon it to his legal injury. Anything calculated to deceive, whether by a single act or combination, or by suppression of truth, or suggestion of what is false, whether it be by direct falsehood or innuendo, by speech or silence, word of mouth, or look or gesture.

Plagiarism is the act of taking or using the ideas or words of another as one's own; the use of someone else's words or documents in such a way as to imply creation and ownership; use of such words, verbatim, without crediting the source; to present as new and original an idea or product known to have been developed or derived from someone else. In writing, the verbatim use of someone else's words without attribution, regardless of intent, is plagiarism, whether the failure to make proper attribution was a careless oversight or intentional.

Falsification is the act of making something false or untrue to deceive, mislead, or misrepresent.

Fabrication is the act of making up or creating to deceive, mislead, or misrepresent. Examples include "back dating," so that a study visit fits within a designated time window and "shaving" numbers from blood pressure readings to meet eligibility criteria for enrollment.*

---

* This definition and the one for plagiarism have been adopted from reference 83.

Acts motivated by deceit, deception, or trickery constitute misconduct. The element of intent is evident in the definitions of fraud, as given above. Even acts of omission can be fraudulent if intended to deceive. (For a scholarly discussion of misconduct in clinical trials see reference 108.)

The usual punishment for persons found guilty of research misconduct is debarment, voluntary or imposed, to exclude them from receiving or participating in federally funded projects and from sitting on federal advisory panels. The debarment is usually for a specified period of time, typically three to five years in cases disposed of by the Office of Research Integrity (ORI).

Institutions receiving federal monies for research must comply with requirements for review and disposition of alleged cases of research misconduct, as set forth in 42 CFR Part 50 (Subpart A: Responsibility of PHS awardee and applicant institutions for dealing with and reporting possible misconduct in science; http://ori.dhhs.gov/misconduct/reg_subpart_a.shtml). Decisions of institutional officials to initiate investigations of alleged cases of misconduct must be reported to the Office of Scientific Integrity (OSI), as well as findings or actions taken on completion or termination of such investigations. The OSI may perform its own investigation as well.

The ORI website (http://ori.dhhs.gov/misconduct/cases/) contains a summary of research misconduct resulting in administrative action by the ORI (limited to the current year and the two preceding years). The list, as of October 13, 2010, named 38 persons. The list includes M.Ds, Ph.Ds, professors, nurses, phlebotomists, postdoctoral students, graduate students, medical students, clinic coordinators, and research assistants.

The predominant finding in cases reviewed by the ORI was falsification and/or fabrication of data. Several findings were related to the publication of falsified data or the use of falsified data in funding applications submitted to the National Institutes of Health. One of the cases involved a clinic coordinator in a multicenter clinical trial.

The U.S. Food and Drug Administration (FDA) maintains a "blacklist" of people it has disqualified or restricted in relation to work or providing services pursuant to developing "evidence to support the safety and effectiveness of investigational drugs (human and animal), biological products, and medical devices." The list of permanent disqualifications includes 114 people (as of December 1, 2008) with the dates they entered the list ranging from 1965 to present (http://www.fda.gov/ora/compliance_ref/bimo/dis_res_assur.htm).

Misconduct in data collection is the act of knowingly recording or entering anything that is false. The likelihood is that no trial is devoid of fraudulent data because isolated acts of data falsification or fabrication are difficult to detect. However, the chance of detection increases with frequency, in the same way that a burglar is more apt to get caught the more burglaries committed.

Data have patterns and interrelationships. It was lack of a relationship that led to the identification of a blood pressure reader in the Hypertension Prevention Trial (HPT)[63] who made up the second of two blood pressure readings on study participants–the second one being done about 30 seconds after the first reading. A comparison of the variances of the paired readings across readers revealed a smaller variance than that for other readers. Investigation and questioning ultimately led to an admission that the reader was making up the second reading.

By and large, people are not smart enough to make up data. For example, the Internal Revenue Service identifies suspicious tax returns by looking at the frequency of terminal digits on returns. Fabricated returns have higher frequencies of 5's and 6's for terminal digits than is the case with legitimate returns (http://www.nctm.org/resources/content.aspx?id=7678).

Variables have expected characteristics. The likelihood of anyone being able to make up data mimicking those characteristics is slim.

Data centers can be expected to monitor data patterns by making comparisons across people performing the same functions and across clinics in multicenter trials. Differences across clinics in the timing of study visits led to suspicions of "back dating" at one clinic in the Study of Ocular Complications of AIDS (SOCA) (http://www.jhucct.com/soca/lsoca/trials.htm). The clinic, when compared with other clinics in the study, had a disproportionate number of visits on the last day of permissible time windows. Suspicions were heightened by a number of visits recorded as having been done on Saturdays and Sundays.

An observation of differences in data patterns across centers for measurements made on dog hearts for a multicenter collaborative animal study triggered an extensive investigation.[11] Data for measurements at one site (the Harvard site) showed a more consistent, less varying pattern than for the other three participating sites. The investigations eventually led to a confession by Harvard investigator John Darsee that he had fabricated the data; he was debarred for a period of ten years.[19]

Occasionally, data come to data centers labeled "false." That was the case for a data form received at the National Surgical Adjuvant and Bowel Project (NSABP) coordinating center from the St Luc Hospital in Montreal. The clinic, under the direction of Roger Poisson, kept two sets of records to keep track of what was reported to the data center and what was the truth. The fabrications and falsifications related primarily to eligibility requirements for enrollment, done to enhance enrollment statistics for the clinic.

The emotional flashpoint came when the *Chicago Tribune* (Sunday March 13, 1994) ran a front-page story with the headline "Fraud in Breast Cancer Study: Doctor Lied on Data for Decade" (by John Crewdson), because it raised the possibility that results published in 1985,[43] indicating that lumpectomy plus radiation was as good as mastectomy, might be wrong. The ensuing brouhaha threatened the entire NSABP and temporarily tarnished the reputation of its chair, Bernard Fisher. Recruitment into NSABP trials fell from 2,318 in April through June of 1993 to 236 in the corresponding quarter a year later.[104] Before the smoke settled, the National Cancer Institute ordered a full audit of records for the trial in question and a reanalysis of its results, excluding patients from the Montreal clinic.[42] Not surprisingly, the conclusion remained unaltered because the clinic accounted for less than 17% of all women enrolled in the trial.

An investigation carried out by ORI found Poisson guilty of having "fabricated or falsified data related to laboratory tests and dates of procedures in 115 separate instances dating from 1977–1990 (*NIH Guide*, Vol. 22, June 23, 25, 1993). He was prohibited from receiving federal grants or contracts, or from sitting on public health advisory committees, boards, or review groups for an eight-year period starting March 30, 1993 and "totally restricted" by the FDA.

There are no tried and true approaches to detecting data fraud. Some come to light through routine monitoring, but there are probably just as many that come to light serendipitously (e.g., as with Poisson), through the complaints of colleagues to higher-ups or to newspaper reporters. The investigation of a case of data fraud in the Multiple Risk Factor Intervention Trial (MRFIT) related to eligibility screening started with a call from someone at the Saint Louis clinic charging data fabrication. The reporters, E.J. Pesberg and L. Timnick, in turn called MRFIT study officials to investigate the allegation. That call triggered an investigation by MRFIT officials, chronicled by Neaton et al.[97] The newspaper story ran on May 3, 1976, in the *Saint Louis Globe-Democrat* over the headline "Federal Investigation into Heart Research Project Here."

There is no way to prevent scientific misconduct by persons bent on such behavior, but the risks can be reduced by study leaders who set high standards for integrity, by establishing and maintaining work environments in which integrity is expected and demanded, and by instructing people engaged in data collection and processing as to their ethical obligations for integrity and of the consequences of misconduct.[116]

The assumption is that people come to trials with built-in ethical standards regarding data collection and processing, but that is not necessarily so. As unthinkable as it may be, one cannot assume people new to medical research come equipped with standards. Education is essential.

11

Myths Regarding Trials

Myths are public dreams, dreams are private myths.

Joseph Campbell

Myths are popular beliefs based on perceptions of reality. We thrive on myths. Maybe they nourish our souls in ways we do not understand. Activities of daily living are driven by myths and misconceptions, many so deep-seated and longstanding that they are accepted as "facts." For example, try to convince someone from Lake Wobegon that it is safer to walk the streets of New York City than Milwaukee or that it is safer to fly than drive.* Facts be damned. You can cite statistics, but they will be greeted, most likely, as warmly as mine when recited to

---

* Based on U.S. Federal Bureau of Investigation (FBI) crime statistics for major U.S. cities, Milwaukee was 17th compared with a rank of 50th for New York City in murders per 100,000 population in 2006 (17.3 vs. 7.3). With regard to travel, data provided by the U.S. Department of Transportation indicated that there were 22 fatalities with U.S. air carriers in 2005 versus 43,400 highway deaths, for rates of 0.3 vs. 1.5 100 million miles traveled, respectively (http://www.bts.gov/publications/national_transportation_statistics/html/table_02_09.html).

my wife. As the quote attributed to Benjamin Disraeli (British statesman; 1804–1881) by Mark Twain reminds us, "There are three kinds of lies: lies, damn lies, and statistics," so when fact versus perception, perception wins.

This chapter deals with some of the myths and misconceptions regarding trials.

Myth 1: Most Trials Are Done with Males

This notion took hold in the 1980s, during the women's liberation movement. It was sparked by a few high-profile, male-only cardiovascular trials undertaken in the late 1960s and '70s.[79] The implication that the National Institutes of Health (NIH) research enterprise was tilted in favor of males gave rise to the Office of Research on Women's Health within the NIH (established in 1990) and to clauses in the NIH Revitalization Act of 1993 requiring

> In the case of any clinical trial in which women or members of minority groups will under subsection (a) be included as subjects, the Director of the NIH shall ensure that the trial is designed and carried out in a manner sufficient to provide for a valid analysis of whether the variables being studied in the trial affect women or members of minority groups, as the case may be, differently than other subjects in the trial.[119]

The "valid" analysis requirement, whether recognized as such by Congress, is a requirement to design trials that are capable of detecting treatment by gender interactions (i.e., whether males and females respond differently to treatment). The mandate, if taken literally, would require trials to be ten times larger than is presently the case. Main effects (differences by treatment group without regard to subgroups) are difficult enough to detect, let alone interaction effects.

Ultimately, the NIH interpreted the requirement to mean an "unbiased assessment" consisting of:

1. Unbiased assignment by gender and racial/ethnic subgroups (e.g., as achieved with randomization),

2. Unbiased assessment of the outcome in study participants, and
3. Use of unbiased statistical analyses and proper methods of inference to estimate and compare the intervention effects among the gender and racial/ethnic subgroups.[51]

The reality is that the evidence supporting the perception that the NIH research enterprise was tilted in favor of males was lacking, save for a few celebrated, large, multicenter, male-only trials (see Chapter 7). For example, in 1990, when the legislation was being considered, the number of female-only trials published was about the same as the number of published male-only trials (Table 11.1).

Table 11.1 Clinical trial and randomized controlled trial as publication types [pt] by gender

	Male and Female	Male-only	Female-only	Female-only/ Male-only
Clinical trial [pt]				
1990	7,177	1,195	1,146	0.96
2007	27,022	2,171	3,545	1.63
Randomized controlled trial [pt]				
1990	4,528	694	721	1.04
2007	13,611	1,204	1,872	1.55

Myth 2: Women and Their Diseases Are Understudied Relative to Those of Males

Understudied relative to what measure? Dollars spent on "female" research versus "male" research? Counts of female-only versus male-only trials? Females versus males in the general population? (See Chapter 2 for comments on the term *understudied*.) The perception is hard to substantiate by any measure (see Chapter 7).

Myth 3: The Validity of Trials Depends on Having Representative Study Populations

Hardly. Validity in randomized trials is internal to the trial. Comparisons are valid if treatment assignment is the most parsimonious explanation of the results. It is the absence of treatment-related biases, ruled out by randomization and other measures, such as masking, to reduce the risk of observer bias.

In reality, there is no way to have a representative population for study. The requirement of consent alone works against that since one cannot study those who do not consent to being studied.

Myth 4: Most People in Trials Are Not Informed of Being in Trials

Not true. Virtually every trial, regardless of where done in the world, requires consent. Investigators and institutional review boards (IRBs) alike go to considerable lengths to try to make certain persons are informed before being enrolled. The consent process, in the case of randomized trials, includes efforts aimed at making certain that persons approached for study understand what the trial is about, the treatments being evaluated, and that the treatment they will receive will be decided by the equivalent of a coin flip.

Myth 5: The Primary Purpose of Randomization Is to Provide Comparable Treatment Groups

Wrong. The main reason is to remove bias from the assignment process. A side benefit is that it provides the basis for certain statistical analyses and tests of significance; but its primary purpose is to provide assignments that are immune from the wishes or desires of patient and investigators alike (see Chapter 2 for more). To be sure, on average, randomization does a good job in providing comparable treatment groups, but comparability is not assured for any given trial.

Myth 6: To Be Valid, a Trial Has to Be Masked

Masking is done to reduce the risk of treatment-related bias. Validity may be adversely affected if treatment-related observer bias occurs (i.e., bias, differential by treatment assignment). However, if the outcome measure of interest is immune to observer error (e.g., as in a trial with mortality as the outcome of interest), the chance of such bias is remote. The more subjective the outcome measure, the greater the importance of masking in protecting the validity of the trial.

Myth 7: Trials Subject to Selection Biases Are Invalid

If that were so there would not be any valid trials because all trials are subject to selection biases. The validity of trials comes from having comparable groups of people for comparison across treatment groups. Comparisons are valid so long as the selection biases are the same across treatment groups, as typically occurs with randomization.

Myth 8: Trials Funded by the United States Government Should Meet Our Ethical Standard Regardless of Where Done

One can make the argument, but it is a form of ethics elitism that implies that we are the ethical beacon of the world when it comes to medical research. There are plenty of reasons to question that view.

This issue came to the fore in the late 1990s, in relation to trials done in Thailand[128] and Uganda[55] involving treatment of HIV-infected pregnant women. They were done to see if lesser doses and schedules of anti-HIV treatment would be as effective as the dosage and schedule of zidovudine (AZT) found to be effective in preventing mother-to-child HIV transmission in a trial done in the United States and France (ACTG protocol 076).[26]

The conclusion in the Uganda trial was: "This simple and inexpensive regimen (nevirapine) could decrease mother-to-child HIV-1 transmission in less-developed countries."[55] But the study was conducted with a suboptimal treatment schedule. That fact led to a firestorm of protests, spearheaded by an editorial in the *New England Journal of Medicine* entitled "Investigators' Responsibility for Human Subjects in Developing Countries,"[7] implying that the trial was unethical, even though it produced results of practical value in the Uganda setting.

Myth 9: Most Clinical Trials Are Done by Drug Companies

Not so. Among the 30,508 English-language publications (count as of July 19, 2008) published in 2007 and indexed to the publication type "clinical trial" by the National Library of Medicine, half (15,827) did not involve U.S. government funds. The corresponding count for randomized controlled trials was 7,767 out of 15,151 randomized controlled trials.

Myth 10: Editors Are Largely to Blame for Publication Bias Because of Their Tendency to Reject Negative Trials

Editors do have to shoulder some of the blame, but the biggest contributors to the bias are investigators who simply fail to write up negative or nil results (see also Chapter 3).

Myth 11: Institutional Review Boards Are the Primary Protectors of Study Subjects

The primary protectors are those doing the study. Protection is up close and personal. Institutional review boards are neither close-up nor endowed with the means and wherewithal necessary for ensuring the protection of persons from harm. That responsibility falls to those doing the studying.

The main function of IRBs is in ensuring that proposed research meets accepted ethical standards, that persons will be properly and adequately informed as to the risks and benefits of being studied, and that the research is designed and conducted in a manner to minimize the risk and "nuisance" of being studied.

The reality is that IRB processes have become increasingly burdened with bureaucratic requirements, leading Fost and Levine, in an article entitled "The Dysregulation of Human Subjects Research" to write:

> "...the increasing focus on minutiae has been distracting IRBs from more important substantative issues. The implementation of the regulations [underlying IRBs] and—even more importantly—the federal and institutional interpretations of the regulations' requirements has gone too far."[48]

Myth 12: Data Can Be Spoiled by Looking

"Just as the Sphinx winks if you look at it too long, so if you perform enough significance tests you are sure to find significance, even when none exists" (Cornfield, 1976).[27] Therein lies the problem for the frequentist statistician reliant on p-values for tests of significance in assessing interim results over the course of a trial. Too many looks and the sphinx is likely to wink. The "fix" for the frequentist is to specify the number of looks allowed before the trial starts; this is done to ensure an interpretable p-value for the assessment of differences at the end of the trial. Jerry Cornfield (an internationally renowned biostatistician, 1912–1979), a "likelihoodist," scoffed at the idea of restricting looks simply as a standard operating procedure to frequentists fixated on p-values. (Indeed, it was that scoffing that led to his coining the phrase, "Pig is pigs and data is data" as a way of underscoring that the information is in the data, not in the p-values of differences.)

Myth 13: A Trial Is Not Valid If the Treatments Groups Are Not Comparable

The baseline composition of the treatment groups is never the same. Hence, the question is whether the differences are large enough to explain the treatment differences observed. Generally, they are not, assuming a scheme of treatment assignment that was free of bias, as occurs with randomization.

In any case, the differences observed will have no role in explaining results if the variables that are "different" are not related to the outcome of interest.

Myth 14: Generalization of Findings from Trials Depends on Having Representative Study Populations

One's willingness to generalize findings to a general population is a matter of judgment. The concepts of "generalizability" and "validity" in the context of trials are different. Generalizability relates to the extent to which conclusions can be reasonably generalized beyond the setting of the trial. Validity relates to comparisons within a trial and to the extent to which treatment differences can be legitimately attributed to the experimental variable—treatment assignment.

The scientific basis for generalizations in clinical research depends on being able to select (sample) persons for study from a defined population. Sampling requires a defined (enumerated) population and a sampling frame for selection of persons for study.

The scientific basis for generalization is lacking in clinical trials (and in virtually all other forms of clinical research) because it is impossible to enumerate study populations, let alone define them (other than in general terms). However, even if enumeration was possible, the scientific basis for generalization would still be lacking because people cannot be randomly selected for study. The persons studied would be unrepresentative of the enumerated population to the degree that persons who consent to be studied are different from those who do not.

All generalizations in clinical research are risky, but the risks are reduced in randomized trials because generalizations are to the effects of treatment. Those effects tend to be robust across spectrums of people, to the extent that they share a common underlying biology. That is to say, a treatment that works can be expected to work across a much wider spectrum of people than the select few studied.

Inferences can be made even to people not represented in trials. For example, if aspirin is shown to be an effective primary or secondary preventative against myocardial infarctions in males, it is reasonable to assume that it will have the same effect when used in females.

Similarly, it is reasonable to assume that tamoxifen, found to be effective in use against breast cancer in women, will also be useful in men with breast cancer. Indeed, the drug was approved by the U.S. Food and Drug Administration for use in males, even though the only studies showing effectiveness were done in women.

Generalizations across the age spectrum are common, especially in regard to children. The reality is that most trials are done in adults (19,803 adults-only vs. 3,022 children-only clinical trials [pt], English-language, humans, 2007; counts as of September 7, 2008). This means, that for many treatments, we have more information on adults than on children. (One reason for that is that, quite properly, we are protective of our children. That being so, it is much more difficult and time consuming to clear trials involving children through IRBs than trials involving adults.) As a result, the approach to dosing medicines when used in kids is to regard them as "little adults," with appropriate reductions in dosages—an approach that has its risks.

Myth 15: Study Populations Can Be Defined from Screening Logs

There is a notion that *screening logs* (lists of people screened for enrollment along with basic descriptive data on them) can be helpful in reducing the risks of generalizations (see Myth 14) by knowing how people enrolled differ from those screened but not enrolled. However, the utility of such logs in this regard is questionable since they are themselves select samples of people willing to be screened.

To be sure, screening logs may have utility in recruitment (e.g., by showing who gets excluded and suggesting revisions of exclusion criteria to increase yield) but not in making generalizations less risky.

Myth 16: There Is an Epidemic of Fraudulent Investigators

Unlikely. Remember when milk came in cardboard cartons with all those pictures of missing kids some years back? Eventually, as you ate your breakfast, you got to thinking there was an epidemic of missing kids. The pictures disappeared when we moved from cardboard to plastic containers for milk, but they have been replaced by an endless parade of Amber Alerts and news stories of missing children.

Surely, there is an epidemic. But the reality is that kids have gone missing as long as we have been around. The Bible is filled with accounts of kidnappings.

In truth, the rate of "lost, injured, or otherwise missing" kids has declined, from 7 per 1,000 children aged 0 through 17 years in 1988 to about half that rate in 1999, as reported by the U.S. Department of Justice, Office of Justice Programs, Office of Juvenile Justice and Delinquency Prevention (http://www.ncjrs.gov/pdffiles1/ojjdp/206179.pdf; accessed July 30, 2008).

Data on documented cases of fraudulent behavior among researchers is harder to come by, but it is difficult to believe that the rate per 1,000 investigators is increasing. The reason for the perception is due, no doubt, in part to the publicity that cases receive in this Information Age and to the fact that there is, perhaps, more "looking" and hence more "finds."

Fraudulent behavior is part of the human condition dating back to when man was still living in caves. It is naive, therefore, to think that somehow persons anointed as "researchers" are immune from the behavior.

In the strictest sense of the term, the adage "show me a research project, and I will show you some fraud" likely applies. Hence, in some sense, the question is not whether, but how much. Further, for every case in all of the sciences that is uncovered, there are probably hundreds, if not thousands that go unnoticed.[116]

Myth 17: Conflicts of Interest Are Commonplace in Trials

Largely false, but there are always enough cases to reinforce the public perception that the statement is true.

Myth 18: The Only Subgroup That Should Be Looked At Are Those Specified Before the Trial Started

Not so. The trialist has a duty, before publishing results, to determine whether the effect observed is homogeneous across subgroups represented in the trial. He or she cannot make that determination without looking at treatment differences by subgroups (see Chapter 17).

Myth 19: Care in Trials Is Substandard

Not likely—if anything, it is more likely to be superior. Investigators have ethical obligations to ensure that people enrolled receive proper care, independent of the treatment groups to which assigned. Hence, as a rule, the assigned treatments are on top of usual care procedures. Institutional review boards are unlikely to allow randomization if treatment is substandard.

The 29th item in the 2000 Helsinki Code (http://www.wma.net/e/policy/b3.htm) specifies that:

The benefits, risks, burdens, and effectiveness of a new method should be tested against those of the best current prophylactic, diagnostic, and therapeutic methods. This does not exclude the use of placebo, or no treatment, in studies where no proven prophylactic, diagnostic, or therapeutic method exists.

Myth 20: Trials Sponsored by Drug Companies Are Suspect Because of Conflicts of Interest

Conflicts of interest are not unique to the drug industry. Academic institutions, if ever immune from conflicts driven by money, are increasingly conflicted by becoming themselves involved in drug development and in patenting drugs and medical devices.[6] The issue is not about conflicts of interest but rather whether they are biasing and the extent to which processes and procedures in the trial are shielded from potentially biasing conflicts of interest.

Clearly, drug companies have investments in trials and hopes for positive results, but there is no financial gain in marketing bad drugs. In fact, in some sense, drug company sponsors are perhaps more sensitive to the need for arms-length arrangements with those doing the trial than other types of sponsors.

By and large, researchers are researchers regardless of who employs them. Even within drug companies, a gulf exists between marketing people and researchers.

Myth 21: People with Conflicts of Interest Should Be Excluded from Roles in Trials

The trouble is that people come with conflicts of interest. Only Alfred E. Newman is devoid of them, so to insist on purity by absence of conflicts of interest is tantamount to eliminating connections to people who, in fact, may be most knowledgeable about the treatments being evaluated.

Myth 22: Treatment Effects Monitoring Committees (aka Data Monitoring Committees) Should Be Masked

Such masking is practiced, but is it a good idea? That depends on who you ask. Those who think it is a good idea say that masking makes monitoring more objective because monitors do not know if the trend they see (if one emerges) is indicative of benefit or harm. But those who think masking is a bad idea (me among them) point out that, as soon as a trend emerges, it is important to know whether the trend is indicative of benefit or harm. If monitors are masked, all they know is that there is a difference, but not its sign.

Masking is predicated on the assumption that decision-making in monitoring is symmetrical. That is to say, the decision to stop or alter a trial is independent of whether the effect is positive or negative; but the reality is that the decision depends on the sign of the difference. In general, one is willing to continue longer in the face of a positive trend than in the face of a negative one.

For arguments against such masking, see a commentary entitled "Masked Monitoring in Clinical Trials: Blind Stupidity?"[82]

Myth 23: Treatment Effects Monitoring Should Be Done with Preordained Stopping Rules

Again, that depends on who you talk to. The world is divided into those who proceed that way and those who do not. The trouble with stopping rules is that they can become blocks to meaningful analysis and discussion, with discussion focused more on whether to stick with the rule than on the results leading to the debate.

In any case, it is difficult to construct rules covering all the eventualities likely to be encountered in trials. Even statisticians who favor rules regard them more as guidelines than as hard and fast rules.

12

Tricks of the Trade from a Cynic

To succeed in life, you need two things: Ignorance and confidence.

Mark Twain

In academia, it is "publish or perish" (sometimes, "publish and perish"). Promotion up the academic ladder, in large measure, depends on publication. The more papers the better, preferably with the candidate as the sole author or, if not sole, then as the first author and with papers in "good" journals.

Most academic institutions have clocks running. Faculty have to progress from assistant, to associate, to full professorship within specified periods of time or it is "curtains." A related important element in promotion is for the candidate to show prowess in bringing research dollars to the candidate's institution through "PIship"—that is, funding awards given to the candidate as the principal investigator (PI).

Now imagine parallel universes, with freshly minted assistant professors, both anxious to "beat the clock." Investigator A associates with a group that aims to undertake a primary prevention trial involving people at risk of developing Alzheimer's disease (AD) to see if nonsteroidal anti-inflammatory drugs (NSAIDs) can prevent the disease. She is excited about the connection, given her conviction that prevention holds the key in the battle against AD, which if unabated, is projected to afflict upward of 5 million people in the United States by mid 2050.[20]

The trial is multicenter, with six clinics, a coordinating center, and an organizational structure that binds the pieces into a working whole. The group agrees that publications coming from the trial will be authored by the Alzheimer's Disease Multicenter Trial Research Group (see Chapter 6 for authorship formats).

Shortly after she joins, and after a couple of unsuccessful attempts, the trial is funded by the National Institutes of Health (NIH) for a five-year period (the maximum allowed under grant funding for any given funding cycle), although it is clear that additional funding will be needed to finish the trial. The trial is designed using AD as the primary out-come measure and is to involve several thousand people randomized to receive one of the two NSAIDs being tested or a matching placebo and a period of treatment and follow-up of at least five years for each person enrolled.

Investigator B charts a different course. She collaborates with an investi-gator funded by drug companies to do phase II trials to assess the safety and efficacy of psychotropic drugs for use in people experiencing cognitive decline. The trials are done in the investigator's clinic and involve 15 to 25 patients per trial. The outcome measure, in all cases, is change in cognitive function, as assessed at entry and at the end of 12 weeks of treatment, using a battery of tests designed to measure cognitive function. Although the issue of authorship did not come up when Investigator B "hired on," it was understood that attri-bution would be of the conventional form, as discussed in Chapter 6.

Now, fast forwarding five years, the trial in universe A just finished recruitment and still has several years to run before it produces publishable results. The only publication produced (authored under the corporate format) is one detailing the design and methods of the trial. Work is under way on a paper describing recruitment procedures in the trial and on another paper detailing the baseline characteristics of the study popula-tion, but these are still months away from submission.

Investigator B has done much better. In the five years since signing on, she has 15 papers to her credit, arising from four trials completed in the interval. In addition, she has three other papers "in press," and among the 18, she is the sole author on one and the first author on four others.

Both Investigator A and B are up for promotion. Investigator B sails through. Investigator A's promotion stalls because she is seen as "nonproductive," and she is ultimately shown the door. Never mind that the information generated by Investigator A's study may be of more public health relevance than that from Investigator B's short-term trials. It is publication that counts!

Clearly, Investigator A could have used a lesson in how to succeed in trials. The antithetical list below is for her benefit, even if too late for her.

1. *Focus on short-term, single-center, trials.* It takes too long to do long-term trials and, hence, much too long before papers are ready to publish. The bell is likely to "toll for thee" before you have enough to show for promotion.

2. *Produce results the world wants to hear.* This rule is a little tricky because, in research, you never know how things will come out. The trouble with results the world does not want to hear is that you can be blamed for the results. After all, if they run counter to prevailing "truths," it must be you that did something wrong, since the world is rarely wrong. Defending yourself against the onslaught of the world can drain your energy and keep you from writing the papers needed for promotion. If you are unlucky enough to be associated with "bad-news" results, your only option is to suffer through the travail, unless, of course, you wimp out and don't publish.

3. *Make certain that, in publications, if you cannot be the sole or first author, you are among the first three authors.* The reasons should be obvious from discussion in Chapter 6 on authorship.

4. *Design trials using surrogate outcome measures rather than "hard" outcomes.* This rule is a corollary of Rule 1. Surrogates are necessary to ensure that trials are short-term.

5. *Do an underpowered trial to show a new treatment is equivalent to an established treatment.* You have to be careful here, especially if the trial is subject to review by the U.S. Food and Drug Administration (FDA). The people there are wise to that game! The advantage to

being underpowered is that the sample is too small to detect the superiority of the established treatment, if indeed it is truly superior. Showing equivalence can earn you points with the sponsor.

6. *Focus on trials likely to produce "good news."* This rule is a cousin of Rule 2. The world loves good news, so if you have some, take advantage of it. If TV networks want to interview you, by all means, do it; the same for newspaper reporters. Even though TV and newspaper interviews do not count as publication, they will certainly increase your aura when being evaluated for promotion.

7. *Data dredge until you find a p-value <0.05 and then report it as an important finding.* The world thrives on "significant" results with p-values of 0.05 or less, especially if they herald "good news" (see Chapter 17 on the art form of data dredging). The trick is not to let on that you dredged the results, hence it is important to convey the impression that the analysis leading to the results was part of your plan from the outset.

8. *Report on a subgroup analysis showing a gender treatment difference, especially if it reinforces the prevailing view that women and their diseases have been understudied.* Those reports are sure to make the news and get you TV and newspaper interviews. There is little downside in reporting what the world knows to be true.

9. *Test a new (and preferably high-tech) treatment and show it to be superior to a current treatment.* The world likes high-tech things. The higher the tech the better. But there is a danger that if the high-tech treatment is a bust, chances are that you could be blamed for the bad news or for having done a "flawed" study. (Hence, it is probably best to stay away from this until you have been promoted.)

10. *Use a composite outcome if the primary outcome does not yield "significant" results.* This rule is a corollary to Rule 7 on data dredging. Just keep combining outcome measures until you find a difference. There must be one lurking about somewhere.

11. *Use laudatory language when writing up your results.* This is important, but you have to be careful not to over do it because the world does not like braggarts. One approach is to use terms like "definitive," "original," "unique," or "landmark" in relation to the trial being reported. But a better way, if you can manage it, is to get someone else to use such terms in relation to your trial and then quote that person.

Other "tricks":

- Consider only "evaluable" patients.
- Ignore events "obviously" not related to treatment.
- Make your primary analysis a "per protocol" analysis.

13

Reading Between the Lines, or How To Read a Journal Article

I can't see the lines I used to think I could read between.

Ogden Nash

Results papers are akin to reference books, not meant to be read like novels, from cover to cover. Indeed, it is likely that the only persons reading them from beginning to end are the authors, referees, and copy editors.

The usual reading order is more or less as shown in Table 13.1. The reading sequence is terminated as soon as the reader has acquired the desired information or determines that the subject matter is uninteresting or that the results are irrelevant to his or her interests or needs.

In everyday life, we usually ignore the "fine print" (often to our lasting regret), but that can be a mistake when reading research papers. For example, a footnote in a paper from the Hypertension Detection and Follow-up Program (HDFP) indicates that:

Because of a systematic error in allocation at one center, 297 of the 11,237 participants have been eliminated from analyses.[62]

Table 13.1 Typical reading order of results papers

Part/section	Reading order
Front page	
Title	1st
Author listing	2nd
Abstract	
Conclusion	3rd
Remainder	4th
Manuscript body	
Introduction	6th
Design and methods	7th
Results	
Text	11th
Tables/figures	5th
Discussion/conclusions	
First paragraph	8th
Last paragraph	9th
Remainder	10th
Back pages	
Reference list	Throughout reading
Credits	With title and author listing
Appendices (if any)	Usually with design/methods section

The "systematic error" was, in fact, data fabrication.

In many ways, the methods section of a results paper is the most important part.* If you want to understand the results, you have to understand how they were generated, and for that, you have to comb through the

---

* Do not be deluded into believing otherwise in journals choosing to save space by using a smaller font for the methods section.

methods section, line by line. But, when reading, you must be as mindful of what is not there as you are of what is there.

Authors are not inclined to tell you what they did not do. You have to infer that from what is not said. For example, you have to infer that the trial is not randomized by absence of the term. Do not expect to read "we report here the results of an unrandomized trial." More likely you will read "we report here the results of an open trial." You have to know that *open* is a euphemism for *unrandomized*, just as you have to know that an *open-label* trial is a euphemism for an *unmasked* trial and that *per protocol analysis* means that the analysis was by treatment received rather than by assigned treatment (intention-to-treat analysis).

The most important words in any paper are the few represented in the title of the manuscript. If carefully constructed, they will tell you something about the design (by use of words such as *randomized, controlled*, and *blind*), something about the disease or condition being treated, and something about the treatments being tested (e.g., *Cardiovascular and Cerebrovascular Results from the Randomized, Controlled Alzheimer's Disease Anti-inflammatory Prevention Trial*[2]).

The second most important words are those in the abstract, which gives the conclusion reached by the study investigators, as in the Alzheimer's Disease Anti-inflammatory Prevention Trial (ADAPT):

> For celecoxib, ADAPT data do not show the same level of risk as those of the APC trial. The data for naproxen, although not definitive, are suggestive of increased cardiovascular and cerebrovascular risk.

So, suppose the paper makes the first cut as relevant and worth a more careful reading? What now? If things are not always the way they seem, how do you read between the lines?

Look for inconsistencies in language or terminology. The difference between a good paper and a bad one is 15 iterations. Usually inconsistencies are either the result of an insufficient number of iterations, or they are purposeful. You have to figure out which. Look for euphemisms, as mentioned above, or telltale words such as "evaluable," as discussed in Chapter 2.

Be suspicious of the motivation of investigators using "gee whiz" graphs (a term coined by Darrell Huff in *How to Lie with Statistics*[60]) to display their results—graphs purposely drawn to accentuate differences by showing only a portion of the graph, without showing the baseline.

Look for "weasel" terms and clauses.* All researchers "weasel" to reflect uncertainty using words like "perhaps," "maybe," and "possibly," and more specific language unique to a field, as with "silent MI" in heart disease to mean a chemical profile consistent with myocardial infarction (MI) but no clinical expression of an MI. Be skeptical of papers in which there is no weaseling, or in which there is too much. Too little indicates too much certainty and too much means lack of certainty.

Other tips for reading between the lines:

1. *How can I tell if the trial was randomized?* You have to depend on what investigators tell you. Be suspicious if they simply say it was randomized without giving any other details. Be suspicious also if they appear to be using the term in a lay sense, as discussed in Chapter 2. Normally, the absence of the term in the title or abstract should be taken as prima facie evidence that the trial was not randomized since investigators are usually proud to display their wares.

2. *How can I tell if the trial was approved by an institutional review board (IRB)?* You should expect to find a statement to that effect somewhere in the paper. However, absence of such a statement should not arouse undue concern as to the ethics of the study since most journals will not publish studies done without IRB approvals.

3. *How can I tell if the trial is registered in clinicaltrials.gov or some other similar register?* In general, you should find the registration number in the abstract of the paper, if registered. However, the fact of registration is only of passing interest in your efforts to read between the lines. The one place where registration may help is in comparing basic information compiled at the registration site with what is in the manuscript.

---

* One of our defects as a nation is a tendency to use what have been called weasel words. When a weasel sucks eggs, the meat is sucked out of the eggs. If you use a weasel word after another there is nothing left of the other. (Theodore Roosevelt, St. Louis, May 31, 1916)

4. *How can I tell if assignments were concealed until release?* The issue of whether assignments remain concealed and unknown to clinic personnel prior to issue (see Chapter 2) is important because the usefulness of randomization as a means of bias control diminishes if people are able to know assignments in advance of being issued. You should expect to find a statement somewhere in the paper indicating how assignments were issued and a description of procedures for ensuring concealment. If such information is not present, you should be suspicious. You can be assured that assignments were not concealed if the authors indicate that assignments were "open." You should be suspicious that concealment was lacking with "envelope schemes" of assignment (schemes in which clinics are provided with numbered, sealed envelopes to be opened as persons are enrolled) in the absence of procedures for ensuring concealment.

5. *How can I tell if treatments were masked?* Investigators will tell you. If they do not mention masking or blinding, you are safe in assuming that treatments were not masked. If investigators mention blinding or masking, they should tell you whether it was single- or double-masked. Be sensitive to qualifiers like "partially double-masked."

6. *How can I tell if masking was effective?* You cannot. You can get some measure of effectiveness by the amount of "unmasking" during the trial, if reported. You get some idea if the masking is merely a facade if the treatments have obvious side-effects that serve to unmask virtually everyone in the trial.

7. *How can I tell what the control/comparison treatment was?* The authors should tell you. The title may tell you (e.g., as in the title *A Randomized, Placebo-controlled Trial of Natalizumab for Relapsing Multiple Sclerosis.*[106]) If the comparison treatment is itself a treatment, it will be designated by some descriptor such as "standard" or "usual," as in *Randomised Controlled Trial of a Short Course of Traditional Acupuncture Compared with Usual Care for Persistent Non-specific Low Back Pain.*[117] If all else fails, read the conclusion.

8. *How can I tell if the results are biased?* You cannot. You can be reasonably certain they are not if the trial was masked and the masking was effective. You can also be reasonably secure they are not if the outcome measure is "hard," not subject to observer bias. You should expect to find some discussion of the possibility of bias in the discussion section in well-written articles.

9. *How can I tell if the analysis is by original treatment assignment?* Authors should tell you how they did the analysis, but mere use of phrases such as "analysis by original treatment assignment" or "analysis by intention to treat," without supporting detail, is not sufficient. You can assume the analysis is not by treatment assignment in the absence of such phrases. As a rule, investigators will not say an analysis is not by treatment assignment but will instead say that they did a *per protocol analysis* (PPA). When you pull the curtain back on that phrase, you will discover the analysis is by treatment administered instead of by treatment assigned.

10. *How can I tell if the primary outcome measure is the one designated as such when the trial was designed?* You may not be able to, unless the paper includes details on sample size calculations done when the trial was designed. You can check the registration site for the trial to see if the outcome measure specified there agrees with the one featured in the paper. This issue is important if the trial finished normally and the results are being reported as positive. The likelihood of "switching" is not great if the results being reported are nil or negative. Also, the issue is irrelevant if the report has to do with a trial that was stopped because of adverse effects.

11. *How can I tell if the paper is ghost written?* You cannot. You can be reasonably sure it is not if the trial was funded by the National Institutes of Health (NIH). The prospect exists (even if rare) with industry-sponsored trials if the results are positive. See reference 33 for a discussion of the concern.

12. *How can I tell who paid for the trial?* Information on sources of funding should be indicated somewhere in the manuscript, typically on the title page or in the credit section.

13. *How can I tell if everybody randomized is accounted for in the primary analyses?* You should be able to tell if the paper has a CONSORT chart.[3] If not, you should be able to tell by cross-checking tables. Discrepancies in denominators from table to table for treatment comparisons are generally an indication that people have been excluded.

14. *How can I tell if the data were dredged?* The giveaway is in the motivation of the investigators, as discussed in Chapter 17. The data dredger is interested in finding small p-values wherever they may exist. Be suspicious if there are conclusions relating to subgroup differences.

15. *How can I tell if investigators have conflicts of interest?* You have to rely on the journal to inform readers of potential conflicts. Most journals have policies requiring disclosure of conflicts of interest.

16. *How can I tell if investigators excluded people from their analyses?* You have to be sensitive to what investigators write. For example if they write, "In this paper, we present results for the 264 evaluable patients studied," you know that they are presenting results for a select group of patients.

14

Critics and Criticisms

Criticism is easier than craftsmanship.

CLM

If you are a consumer of information from trials, you must be able to size up the critics and criticisms of trials. There is no perfect trial. Hence, every trial is subject to criticism, so the issue is not whether or not there are criticisms, but rather what to make of them. The fundamental question always is whether the criticisms are sufficient to cause you to doubt or dismiss the results.

Broadly, critics fall into three general types:

- **Clever critics:** Those who like to play to the gallery by "turning a phrase" at the investigators expense; these tend to deal in broad generalities.
- **Pontifical critics:** Those who have a propensity to be "preachy" and "righteous"; these are likely to question the ethics underlying the trial and to impugn by innuendo.
- **"Joe Friday" critics:** After the fictional lead detective in the long-running radio and TV series *Dragnet*, Joe was the guy with the dry

demeanor and interest only in the facts when interviewing witnesses: "Just the facts ma'am, just the facts." These critics tend to focus primarily on issues of design and conduct likely to impact on the validity of results.

Of the three types, the "Joe Friday" type is the least interesting to watch or read, but the type that deserves the most attention.

You have to be careful about relying on critics of any type when forming your opinion regarding a set of results. Surely, you have been to movies that you enjoyed but that critics hated. In truth, you cannot even be sure that a person holding forth on a trial has even read the paper containing the results being criticized. The person may be a "second-hand critic," using the Chicken Little method of communication.

Some years after my sojourn in the University Group Diabetes Program, I was at a meeting of august advisors. Midway through the meeting, one of the participants rose to hold forth as to what was wrong with the study and how stupid the investigators were, oblivious of my association with the trial.

I listened quietly until he finished and then rose to say, "You have a lot to say about the study. So let me ask you a question? Have you read the paper describing the results?" He admitted that he had not. Whereupon I suggested, "How about a deal? I'll send you a copy of the paper and you read it. After that, you can say whatever you please about the study." I did as I suggested when I got back home but as to whether it changed his view? I have no way of knowing because our paths never crossed again.

There is nothing like the genuine article in forming your opinion. In movies, the "proof" is in the watching; in papers, the proof is in the reading.

So, without the genuine article—the paper reporting the results—you should take all criticisms you hear or read with a grain of salt.

So, how do you get the genuine article? First, you need to know if there is indeed a genuine article. Lots of things bantered in the press and commented upon by critics will be from unpublished preliminary results presented at meetings. If there is no publication, ignore the criticisms.

But suppose the results are published. How do I get the paper? If the research was funded by the National Institutes of Health (NIH) and deposited in PubMed Central (a free digital database of published papers maintained by the National Library of Medicine), you can download a PDF version of the paper to your computer, free of charge.

Some online journals allow free access to their articles, for example, as with PLoS (Public Library of Science) publications. So, if it turns out that you were interested in reading a paper on the cardiovascular and cerebrovascular results from Alzheimer's Disease Anti-inflammatory Prevention Trial (ADAPT)[2] in PLoS, you would be able to download it if you entered the author's name (the ADAPT Research Group). You would be presented with it and two commentaries stimulated by the publication of the article in question.

But, suppose you want to see the ADAPT paper published in *Neurology*?[1] Again, the author is the ADAPT Research Group. The title is "Naproxen and Celecoxib Do Not Prevent AD in Early Results from a Randomized Controlled Trial" (*Neurology* 2007;68:1800–1808). You can try PubMed, but the full-text article isn't stored there; the only thing you will be able to download from PubMed is an abstract of the paper. Unless you belong to an institution with a free downloading license agreement of journal articles, to see the full-text article, you'll have to pay a downloading charge.

Now, assuming that, by hook or crook, you have gotten a copy of the paper and you have read it. What are the things you should worry about?

Pay attention to those things that raise possibilities that the results are not valid because of poor design, conduct, or analysis procedures. (For a catalog of criticisms leveled at the University Group Diabetes Program (UGDP) and answers to them, see Chapter 7 and reference 84.) Those will have to do with the system of assigning people to treatment, and whether the assignment procedure was free of selection bias (as defined in Chapter 2), the outcome measure and its clinical relevance, the possibility that the results can be explained by bias of one kind or another, the adequacy of the sample size and length of follow-up for the question at issue, and whether the analysis is kosher.

Largely, the only criticisms of any value in such assessments will be those published in peer-reviewed indexed literature. Talk is cheap. It takes money to buy whiskey, and unless one is willing to commit criticisms to peer review, they need to be viewed with skepticism.

The questions of relevance are listed in the *Rating Index for Clinical Trials* (Appendix B). The list below details criticisms that you can ignore, being "universal criticisms," if you will, that apply to any trial and, hence, should be viewed with a jaundiced eye unless supported by the facts.

1. *The study is flawed.* This is a favorite of people who do not like the results and want to dismiss them. The statement is vacuous in the absence of substantiated fact. Of course the trial is flawed. Nature abhors perfection. There is no perfect trial. The question is whether the flaws are sufficient to make you doubt the results. If the "flawing" is uniform across treatment groups, all it does is add to noise in the comparison since the comparison of interest is a difference of one treatment group compared to another. So long as the "flawing" is the same across treatment groups, it subtracts out by the differencing process necessary in comparing treatment groups within the trial.

2. *More research is needed.* This is the standard closing sentence of most authors, so it is no surprise that it is high on the list of universal criticisms of critics. The only difference is that often, when used by critics, it is used to suggest that the investigators "blew it" and that they or some other group should go back to the drawing board and do a "decent" trial.

3. *The study is unethical.* This is the trump card of the pontifical critic. If everything else fails, question the ethical underpinning of the trial, or even the ethics of the investigators (although the latter is more dangerous than questioning the underlying ethics of the trial).

4. *The results are open to question because of conflicts of interest.* The world is filled with conflicts of interest, so clever and pontifical critics can raise the concern by innuendo without facts per se. Basically, the criticism arises only when the results reported are positive or negative. It does not normally come up when the results are nil. The issue of the biasing effect of funding may arise

when the trial is industry-sponsored and positive. If it is to have substance, it should be supported by facts.

5. *The investigators studied the wrong population.* This one always works since it is impossible to define the "right" study population. The issue is largely irrelevant in trials producing positive or negative results since, however "wrong" the population may be, it is "wrong" to the same degree for all study groups in randomized trials and hence still provides a valid basis for comparison.

6. *The study population is select.* Of course. Every study population is select for a host of reasons, starting with the requirement that one can only study those who consent to being studied. But as in criticism 5, if the selection is the same across treatment groups, the issue is largely irrelevant.

7. *The study population is not representative of the general patient population.* This one works in any trial. The statement usually means that "the patients are not like the ones I see." The issue is largely irrelevant in randomized trials because if a treatment has an effect, that effect is generally present across a wide spectrum of people.

8. *The study groups are not comparable.* Generally a vacuous criticism; groups are never 100% comparable (see Chapter 2). The question is whether this lack of comparability is sufficient to explain the difference observed; usually, this is not the case.

9. *The treatment difference is explained by baseline differences in the composition of the treatment groups.* Vacuous without supporting analyses to support the criticism.

10. *The difference observed is concentrated in a particular subgroup of patients and hence the authors conclusion should be ignored.* If a critic wants to cast doubt on the authors' overall conclusion regarding a treatment effect, they can resort to the "subgroup argument" — that the difference is isolated to a subgroup of people that accounts for the difference reported. A claim easy to make, but hard to substantiate, so be wary of the argument (see Chapter 17).

11. *Important baseline data, not collected, are likely to explain the results.* Clever, but not usually a criticism of substance. There is

no reason to believe that baseline data not collected will be any more meaningful in explaining results than those collected. Be wary of arguments that there exists some baseline variable (e.g., smoking history in a heart study with a treatment difference), that, although not recorded, is somehow so maldistributed by treatment group that had it been observed and used to adjust results, the difference observed would have disappeared. There is no reason to believe that baseline variables not observed will be distributed any differently by treatment group than those observed. There are always "important data" overlooked, even if trialists are guilty of collecting ten times more data than they need. The question is whether the data not collected will explain away the results. Not likely.

12. *The treatment dose or administration schedule is not like that used in ordinary practice.* All trials are approximations to reality and hence involve compromises. An issue raised in criticisms of the UGDP tolbutamide results was that the trial involved a fixed dose of tolbutamide when in fact, in real life, the dose is varied to achieve the desired blood sugar control. True, but the reality in the trial was that the higher the dose the greater the evidence of ill-effects. Hence, the argument was largely irrelevant in "explaining away" the increased mortality for people on tolbutamide.

15

What to Make of Results

However beautiful the strategy, you should occasionally look at the results.

Winston Churchill

"Pigs is pigs and data is data."* The expression is attributed to Cornfield[28]—a likelihoodist. It was his way of reminding people that the information is in the data, not in the p-values they produce. Most "results" are delivered to us via TV in five-second time slices. If TV is your primary means of monitoring for results of relevance to you, you will be limited largely to results heralding evidence of benefit or harm for

---

* The expression comes from a children's story *Pigs is Pigs* by Ellis Parker Butler (1905)–a story about a dispute over a freight charge. A man orders a pair of guinea pigs for his son, but troubles arise when he arrives at the freight station to pick them up. The railroad agent wants to charge 30 cents apiece for "livestock," but the boy's father argues the charge should be 25 cents for "domestic pets." They deadlocked. The railroad agent refuses to turn the shipment over until the dispute can be settled by higher ups. Weeks turn into months. Eventually, the railroad agent relents, but only after being knee-deep in guinea pigs.

The fact that it is improper English makes the expression even more appealing to one who feels compelled to "correct" students whenever they use *data* as a singular.

common conditions and diseases. The chance of making the news diminishes with the profile of the disease or numbers affected by it. Also, keep in mind that the chance of making the news is significantly increased if the results are even slightly suggestive of treatment-by-gender interactions or differences by ethnic origin.

Suppose, however, a report comes to your attention, and it is about something of interest to you and you want to know how the trial underlying the report was done in order to decide whether you should believe the results. If you are serious, you will have to do some hunting and some work.

One of the first classes I took, after I wandered off the farm into the University of Minnesota, was "Introduction to Chemistry." It was taught by a modestly rotund, five-foot eight-inch, balding professor with an irritatingly high-pitched voice that got two octaves higher whenever he was excited or irritated. The auditorium was filled to capacity with 200-plus students. It was the wake-up 8:30 AM–9:20 AM, MWF course, with chalk flying by 8:31 AM.

Every now and again, there would be some poor soul with courage enough to ask a question about something scribbled on the board. The professor would listen, and if he thought the question was about something the student should know or should have learned from studying (most of the time), he would stare at the poor soul for a few seconds and then, in his highest-pitched, most arrogant tone, would simply say, "Well! There is no royal road to learning!" and turn back to producing chalk dust.

And so it is. Learning is a highly personal effort. It is you versus you.

Your first task is to track down the scientific paper leading to the story. That will take leg work, because news media organizations, especially radio and TV, are not in the habit of laying Hansel and Gretel paths to the original source. But, if you have an author's name, you can Google. You can look for the published results in PubMed and PubMed Central, as discussed in Chapter 14, or in www.clinicaltrials.gov or similar registries.

But there may not be any publication at all. A fair number of medical "discoveries" making the news are from presentations at scientific meetings and conferences prior to any publication. It would be a better, less cluttered world if there was a rule that the results of trials are not presented until they have been published in peer-reviewed journals, but that won't happen. Everybody wants "new," so it is hard to get on programs of major meetings unless you have something new and not yet published.

The very first trial on which I cut my teeth got under way while I was still in graduate school—the University Group Diabetes Program (UGDP).[130] The UGDP was a randomized, multicenter trial designed to test, among other treatments, whether tolbutamide (Orinase), as compared to placebo, was useful in prolonging lives and reducing the long-term complications of type 2 diabetes.

Investigators at the outset of data collection agreed on a "publish first, present later" policy in regard to primary results coming from the trial.

Several years later, in 1969, investigators decided to stop use of tolbutamide in the trial because of a mortality difference against tolbutamide.[130] Accordingly, investigators proceeded to write up the results and submitted them to *Diabetes* in early 1970. But, as often happens with "publish first, present later" policies, investigators looked for "work-arounds," so that they could have their cake and eat it, too.

They wanted to present the results at the annual meeting of the American Diabetes Association (ADA) in St. Louis in mid-June of 1970. They reasoned that the paper, submitted months earlier, would be published by the time of the meeting or within days after. So, they submitted the results for presentation, reasonably sure that their policy would remain intact.

But editors march to their own tune, and publication was not until November. To make the information gap worse, there was a flurry of publicity weeks in advance of the meeting. Unbeknownst to the investigators, the ADA had a policy of providing the press with newsworthy abstracts in advance of the meeting.

The first place the results appeared was on the Dow Jones ticker tape, on May 20 (not surprising, seeing as tolbutamide was a blockbuster drug of Upjohn), followed, in short order, by newspaper stories around the country informing readers that a widely prescribed antidiabetes drug may be causing deaths. Diabetologists were deluged with calls from worried patients as to whether they were on the "killer drug" they were reading about. They were forced to address concerns without benefit of a published paper describing the trial and its results.

Within months of the meeting, the Committee for the Care of the Diabetic (CCD) was formed as a bulwark against the UGDP and the

U.S. Food and Drug Administration (FDA)'s effort to include a warning regarding the possibility of cardiovascular risks associated with the drug, officially proposed in June 1971. It would be 13 years before the labeling change was implemented (March 1984).[84]

The CCD was convinced that there had to be something wrong with the way in which data were analyzed because the results did not jibe with "clinical observation." Ultimately, they requested raw data from the trial's coordinating center under the Freedom of Information Act (FOIA), so that they could do their own analyses.

The court case for the request and a FOIA court case for Henry Kissinger's telephone logs (U.S. Secretary of State) coalesced to be heard together in front of the U.S. Supreme Court in the fall of 1979 and was decided March 1980. (The Court, in a 6 to 2 decision, ruled it was not the intent of Congress for the FOIA to extend to the UGDP or Kissinger's telephone logs, forever linking the UGDP and Henry Kissinger.[121])

But I digress.

If your hunt comes up empty, it is likely that the results being bantered about have not been published. Stand down. Do not make anything of what you have read or heard until there is a published paper.

Suppose you come up with the paper. Now, do you have data that you need to evaluate the results? Maybe, maybe not. You are looking at "filtered" results; filtering due to what investigators choose to publish and what editors will publish.

It is said that, in making a movie, 90% of the film falls on the cutting room floor. The same is true of manuscripts. Well-written ones go through a half-dozen or more iterations from start to submission and a couple more after submission to acceptance. Hence, lots of analyses and tables produced along the way never make it into the finished paper.

There is no such thing as unfiltered information, even if you sat in the data center for the trial. Data are "edited" and "cleaned" before they are analyzed; edited to check for inconsistent information, imputation of missing data, and "trimming" to reduce the influence of extreme values on distribution dependent statistics. The hope you have as a reader is that the filtering is independent of the treatment results.

The first question you have to answer, with a paper in hand is: Are the results relevant to my interests or needs? That requires a *relevance assessment*, as represented by question below from the *Rating Index for Clinical Trials* (see Appendix B).

A Clinical Relevance Index

Cumulative scores range from 5 to 21. If the score is high, proceed; if ≤10 look for some other trial more relevant to your interest or condition.

Score Sum

1. Primary outcome measure? (see Chapter 3) ____ ____
   3 Clinical event
   2 Surrogate outcome measure
   1 Change measure
   0 Not specified

2. Clinical relevance of outcome measure to condition
   of interest? ____ ____
   3 High
   2 Intermediate
   1 Low

3. Eligibility and exclusion criteria appropriate? ____ ____
   3 Yes
   0 No

4. Eligibility requirements relevant to my condition? ____ ____
   3 Yes
   0 No

5. "Real-world" treatment regimen? ____ ____
   3 Closely parallels real-world regimen
   2 Modestly parallel to real-world regimen
   1 Remotely related to real-world regimen

Score Sum

6. Place of conduct?   ____ ____
   2 Similar to where I would go for care
   1 Not similar to where I would go for care

7. Period of treatment?   ____ ____
   2 Period of treatment sufficient to assess safety
      and efficacy of treatment
   1 Period of treatment too short to reliably assess safety
      and efficacy

8. Period of follow-up?   ____ ____
   2 Period sufficient to assess safety and efficacy of
      treatment
   1 Period not sufficient to assess safety and efficacy

Next, you need to assess your level of skepticism regarding the results, as assessed by completing the Skepticism Index, below. The lowest skepticism score possible is 0, but in all likelihood, not many trials will yield that score. Therefore, you probably should be satisfied with scores below 10.

Skepticism Index

Keep a running score as you proceed. If at any time it is 30 or higher, your level of skepticism is probably too high for you to have faith in the results. Try to find another trial yielding a lower skepticism score.

Score Sum

1. Where published?   ____ ____
   30 Self-published
   25 Throwaway medical journal
   10 Newspaper/news stand magazine
    5 Book/monograph/meeting proceedings
    5 Medical journal, not National Library of
       Medicine -indexed (i.e., not in PubMed)
    0 Medical journal, in PubMed

Score Sum

2. Published in a major, high-circulation, medical journal?   ____ ____
   3 No
   0 Yes

3. Authorship format? (see Chapter 6)   ____ ____
   30 No authorship attribution
   15 Byline
   2 Conventional
   1 Modified conventional
   0 Corporate

4. Institutional affiliation of investigators provided?   ____ ____
   15 No
   0 Yes

5. Sponsorship?   ____ ____
   15 Not stated
   2 Drug company/for profit business
   1 Nonprofit foundation
   0 NIH/Governmental agency

6. Site of conduct?   ____ ____
   3 Single site (single-center)
   0 Multiple sites (multicenter)

7. Purpose of trial?   ____ ____
   15 Not stated/cannot determine
   2 Noninferiority (to show test treatment is not worse than comparator treatment)
   2 Equivalence (to show test treatment is equivalent to comparator treatment)
   0 Superiority (to show test treatment is superior to comparator treatment)
   2 Other

Score Sum

8. Reason for publication?   ____ ____
   15 Not stated/cannot determine
   5 Interim report (trial still continuing;
     no major change in the study
     protocol)
   0 Early stop of trial because of evidence
     of benefit or harm (see Chapter 2)
   0 Normal end (trial went to scheduled end)

9. Comparison group?   ____ ____
   5 None
   5 External/historical control
     (see Chapter 1)
   0 Internal (concurrently enrolled and
     followed)

10. Treatment groups?   ____ ____
    5 One
    0 Two or more (including control treatment)

11. Mode of treatment assignment?
    (see discussion in Chapter 2)   ____ ____
    25 Only one treatment group
    25 Patient/physician choice
    15 Systematic (e.g., odd days to test treatment;
       even days to control treatment)
    15 Open "random" (e.g., test treatment
       if last digit of hospital record odd; control
       treatment if even)
    5 Concealed "random"; claimed but
      insufficient detail to determine
    0 Concealed random; detailed

12. Primary outcome measure specified?   ____ ____
    10 No
    0 Yes

Score Sum

13. Risk of bias in primary outcome? ____ ____
    10 Primary outcome not specified/cannot determine
    7 High (unmasked and subjective measure)
    3 Low (double-masked and subjective measure)
    0 Nil (objective measure like death or laboratory test)

14. Masking? ____ ____
    2 None
    1 Single
    0 Double

15. CONSORT-like chart or table giving numbers enrolled and followed?[3] ____ ____
    30 No
    0 Yes

16. Rationale for sample size stated? ____ ____
    20 No
    0 Yes

17. Sample size adequate for conclusions reached? ____ ____
    30 No
    15 Uncertain
    0 Yes

18. Study participants followed regardless of compliance to treatment? ____ ____
    30 No
    15 Uncertain
    0 Yes

19. Analysis limited to "evaluable" patients? ____ ____
    30 Yes
    15 Uncertain
    0 No

If the skepticism score is low enough, you should move on to the Analysis Confidence Index. The questions here have to do with issues of counting, whether the analysis was by treatment assignment (intention-to-treat), and with the sophistication of the authors in interpreting their results. The highest possible score is 150. Scores near zero or negative are bad news.

Analysis and Discussion Confidence Index

Score Sum

1. All persons assessed for outcome regardless of
   adherence to treatment?
   15 Yes
    0 Cannot determine
   –5 No

2. All outcome events counted from moment of
   enrollment forward in time?
   15 Yes
    0 Cannot determine
   –5 No

3. All persons counted to treatment group to
   which assigned?
   15 Yes
    0 No/Cannot determine

4. Are the conclusions supported by the data?
   15 Yes
    0 No

5. Is the conclusion about a subgroup effect or
   interaction?
   15 No
    5 Yes

Score Sum

6. Subgroup analyses to assess homogeneity of
treatment effect?   ____ ____
   15 Yes
    0 No/uncertain

7. Dredged subgroup difference? (see Chapter 17)   ____ ____
   15 No
    0 Uncertain
   –10 Yes

8. Is the treatment effect homogeneous across
subgroups? (see Chapter 17)   ____ ____
   10 Yes
    0 No

9. Discussion or presentation of side effect data?   ____ ____
   15 Yes
    0 No

10. Are p-values used as indicators of truth?
(see Chapter 16)   ____ ____
   15 No
   –5 Yes

11. Discussion including summary of relevant
previous studies and trials?   ____ ____
    5 Yes
    0 No

12. Discussion of strengths, weakness, and limitations
of trial?   ____ ____
    5 Yes
   –5 No

If the clinical relevance is high, your level of skepticism low, and your confidence in the analysis high, you are ready for the coup de grâce questions below. If the cumulative score for these questions goes negative, you are well advised to ignore the results.

The granddaddy question is the last one: *Do I believe the results are reproducible?* If you do—i.e., that others doing a similar trial would get the same results—then you should believe the results, regardless of the p-value affixed to them. If you do not, you should not be influenced by p-values, regardless of how small.

The Coup de Grâce Questions

Score Sum

1. Do I trust the investigators?
   5 Yes
   0 No

2. Do I believe the results?
   5 Yes
   0 No

3. Do I think the results have been dredged to
   find a "significant" difference?
   5 No
   0 Yes

4. Do I believe the results are reproducible?
   5 Yes
   0 No

Good luck!

16

Biostatistics 101

Facts are stubborn things, but statistics are more pliable.

Mark Twain

Chances are that most readers of this book will have had a course in biostatistics. Hence, the purpose here is simply to provide a refresher, specific to clinical trials, and a glossary of terms and definitions relevant to the analyses of clinical trials.

The question, in the class of trials considered here (superiority, randomized phase III or IV trials with parallel-treatment designs), is whether the results are sufficient to conclude that the test treatment is superior to the comparison control treatment. The approach in addressing the question depends on the school of thought guiding the analysis, broadly:

- Bayesian
- Likelihood
- Frequentist

Staunch members of these schools are like religious sects, each claiming to be members of the one true school and scoffing at members of the other schools. Reasons for the differences are beyond this review, save to say that all three approaches have merits and shortcomings.

However, although the schools of thought provide different frameworks for statistical inference, members of all three schools subscribe to the basic rules of counting and analysis as put forth in Chapter 3. Hence, this refresher is predicated on an underlying understanding of those rules.

The focus here is from the frequentist perspective. Almost all of the inferences in papers from the class of trials considered are from that perspective, as evidenced by mentions of significance tests, p-values, and confidence intervals in published papers from trials.

The frequentist perspective is hypothesis-based. Broadly, from this perspective, a trial is seen as a test of two hypotheses, the *null hypothesis* of no difference in effect between the test and control treatment and a *one-tailed alternative* that the test treatment is better than the control treatment or a *two-tailed alternative* that the test treatment is better or worse than the control treatment. Sample size calculations are made against specified type I error (probability of rejecting the null hypothesis when it is true) and type II error (probability of accepting the null hypothesis when it is false).

The primary analysis centers on whether to accept or reject the null hypothesis; in simplest terms, this is done by a test of significance and the resulting p-value to judge statistical significance. If the p-value is not appropriately small (say, >0.05), the null hypothesis is accepted and the conclusion is that test treatment is no better or worse than the control treatment.

If the p-value is appropriately small (say, ≤ 0.05), the null hypothesis is rejected and the alternative hypothesis is accepted. The inference as to whether the test treatment is better or worse than the control treatment depends on the sign of the treatment difference. The inference is that the test treatment is better than the control treatment if the difference is positive. If it is negative, the inference is that the test treatment is worse than the control treatment.

Obviously, conclusions represented in papers are inferences because there is no way to know, with certainty, if the null hypothesis is true or false. The p-value is the proportion of times one would expect to observe a p-value as extreme or more extreme than the one observed if the null hypothesis is, in fact, true and the trial in question is repeated many times under conditions identical to the trial in question. Hence, a p-value, no matter how small, does not mean that the null hypothesis is false. It simply means that the p-value is consistent with it being false.

Inference from a single trial regarding the truth of a hypothesis is like concluding that a coin that comes up heads in a single toss is a coin with heads on both sides. The risk of being wrong in a single trial is sizable. That is why the need exists for "re-search," as discussed in Chapter 19.

Readers will see results summarized by p-values or by confidence intervals in results papers from trials. Confidence intervals are for estimates, and p-values are for tests of significance. Consider the results presented in Table 17.1 in Chapter 17. The treatment effect measured by the difference in proportion dead in the two treatment groups is exactly 0.0. The 95% confidence interval about the estimate is –0.14 to +0.14.

Ninety-five percent confidence estimates that include the value zero correspond to p-values of greater than 0.05. Intervals that do not include that value correspond to p-values that are less than 0.05.

If the choice is between p-values and confidence intervals for characterizing results from trials, the choice should be confidence intervals. They are more informative and preferred by journal editors.[54,86]

In reality, however, the actual process of analysis and inference is considerably more complicated than merely testing a hypothesis and deciding whether to accept or reject it. First, investigators have to be satisfied that their analysis and conclusions are valid. For openers, they have to be satisfied that tests performed are valid. All tests of significance involve assumptions regarding the underlying data, assumptions that are typically violated to varying degrees. Tests vary as to robustness against departures from the assumptions. The question for investigators is whether the departures are serious enough to invalidate the test and, hence, their conclusions.

Second, investigators need to determine whether their results are confounded by differences in the baseline composition of the treatment groups. If there are big differences in composition, the possibility exists that the difference, rather than treatment assignment, accounts for the observed treatment differences. Although big differences are unlikely in randomized trials, the reality is that randomization does not rule out the possibility of baseline differences. The usual approach in answering the question to one's self and readers' satisfaction is to compare crude (unadjusted) results with results adjusted for baseline differences. If the crude and adjusted results are about the same, the conclusion is that the treatment difference is not explained by baseline differences. If they differ markedly, then the treatment effect is questionable.

Another question that investigators have to address is whether the treatment effect is homogeneous—that is, is the same across subgroups represented in the trial. Does the inference apply across the spectrum of patients studied, or only to a subgroup? Readers should expect to see some evidence of the issue having been addressed, typically by subgroup analyses (see Chapter 17 for discussion).

In the ideal trial, every person randomized receives the assigned treatment, is 100% compliant with the treatment, and is followed exactly as required by the study protocol. In the ideal world, there is no censoring, except for the uninformative censoring related to when people are enrolled (see definition below). But in the real world, there are missed visits, dropouts, and less-than-perfect treatment compliance. If any of these measures are differential by treatment group (likely), the treatment comparisons may be biased because of the censoring. Hence, the analysis has to address the question as to whether the differences are due to informative censoring.

Glossary of Statistical Terms

- **adjusted data**—Data subjected to an **adjustment procedure**; the opposite of **unadjusted data**.
- **adjustment procedure**—Any of a variety of procedures intended to remove the effect of one or more extraneous sources of variation affecting a result; in trials, procedures include **subgroup analysis**, analysis of covariance, and regression analysis involving baseline characteristics.
- **alternative hypothesis**—1. A hypothesis stated as an alternative to the **null hypothesis**, in which parameters in the hypothesis are

assigned non-null values. 2. The hypothesis that is accepted when the null hypothesis is rejected. See also: **one-tailed alternative hypothesis; two-tailed alternative hypothesis.**

- **analysis by assigned treatment**—Data analysis in which persons are counted to the treatment group to which assigned, regardless of compliance to the treatment; required for **intention-to-treat analysis.**

- **Bayesian**—Being or relating to a school of thought in which a prior probability distribution is assigned to parameters by application of Bayes' theorem. The resulting posterior probabilities are viewed as measures of existing evidence. See also: **frequentist, likelihoodist.**

- **Bayesian analysis**—Any method of data analysis in which prior information or belief concerning some condition (expressed in the form of a prior probability distribution) is used in conjunction with data obtained from a study or experiment (expressed in the form of a likelihood function) to draw inferences concerning the condition. See also: **Bayesian, frequentist, likelihoodist.**

- **censor, censored, censoring, censors**—Broadly, to delete, suppress, or eliminate. *Usage note*: In the context of trials, censoring occurs when an observation cannot be made or is not counted in an analysis because of some intervening condition or event, or when not made available in an effort to preserve treatment masking. An example of the latter type of censoring is when laboratory determinations are withheld from clinic personnel in masked trials because of concern that, if known to them, the information may unmask treatments. Most censoring is of the former kind and arises from the fact that enrollment continues over a period of time, and therefore persons at any point in time during the trial are seen for differing periods of time, depending on when enrolled. For example, suppose observation up to January 30, 1996, for an interim analysis, one person enrolled on November 30, 1995 (P_1) and one person enrolled on December 30, 1995 (P_2). P_1 contributes 61 person-days and P_2 contributes 31 person-days of observation. Observation of P_2 beyond day 31 is censored because of when enrollment occurred. A second form of censoring occurs because of missed visits or dropouts. For example, suppose it is not possible to observe P_1 beyond day 45 because the person refused further observation. Observation is censored at day 45 for variables requiring a compliant person for observation. Both forms of censoring arise from inability or failure to observe. Another form arises from eliminating observations made after the occurrence of some event or condition. For example, suppose an analysis involving the comparison of treatment groups for an event (e.g., the first occurrence of systolic blood pressure above a specified level) while on assigned treatment. Suppose that P_2 was taken off assigned treatment on day 15 and that the event of interest occurred on day 20. Observation, for purposes of the analysis, would be censored at day 15 and the event, although observed, would not be counted. Censoring not related to the variable of interest is referred to as *uninformative censoring* (e.g., the censoring in the first example). Censoring related to the measure or event of interest is referred to as *informative censoring* (e.g., censoring in the second example, if missed visits are treatment-related).

- **confidence interval**—An interval of values estimated from observed data presumed to include the parameter of interest (e.g., the **treatment difference**) at a specified confidence level. For example, the 95% confidence interval for the observed mean, x, of a normally distributed variable, estimated from a sample drawn from a larger underlying population, is centered at x and has a lower endpoint of $x - 1.96 \cdot SE_{(mean)}$ and an upper end point of $x + 1.96 \cdot SE_{(mean)}$. Ninety-five percent of such intervals, constructed from independent samples from the larger underlying population, will contain the true population mean (parameter). However, there is no assurance that any given interval will do so. Typically, the interval is defined by both a lower and upper endpoint, but it will have just one endpoint if the **type I error** represented in the **confidence level** is one-tailed.

- **confidence level**—One minus the specified **type I error** level for a **confidence interval**; often multiplied by 100 to express as a percent.

- **confounding variable**—1. In epidemiology, broadly, a variable, causally related to some outcome, that distorts an association between that outcome and some precursor event or exposure by obscuring or falsely accentuating the association. Defined by Last[71] as "A variable that can cause or prevent the outcome of interest, is not an intermediate variable, and is associated with the factor under investigation." 2. In trials, any variable, observed before or on enrollment, related to treatment assignment or that, by chance, is related to treatment assignment and that influences outcome; e.g., a baseline variable differentially distributed among the treatment groups that is related to outcome. *Usage note*: It is important to distinguish between variables observed before treatment assignment and those observed after assignment. Variables of the former kind, by definition, are independent of treatment assignment, whereas variables of the latter kind may not be. The distinction is important in that variables of the former kind may help explain the size, presence, or absence of a treatment difference, whereas variables of the latter kind may themselves be confounded with treatment and therefore cannot explain a treatment difference. For example, compliance measures, by definition observed after the initiation of treatment, may help explain how a treatment works but cannot explain a **treatment difference**.
- **control variable**—An independent variable **controlled** in analysis by adjustment or stratification.
- **controlled**—1. Any system of observation and data collection designed to provide a basis for comparing one treatment group with another, such as provided in a parallel-treatment design with concurrent enrollment to the study groups represented in the design. 2. Data analysis involving use of control variables. *Usage note*: Often unnecessary or redundant as a modifier, especially as a modifier of design terms that, in and of themselves, convey the notion of control, as in *randomized **controlled** trial* (the modifier randomized indicates the nature of the control implied). Often redundant in the broader setting of trials as well, even if not randomized, since the notion of control is usually implicit in such usages.

One can assume that the notion of control applies in all research settings involving experimentation. However, it is conventional to use the term as a modifier of a trial, especially when not preceded or followed by the modifier *randomized.*

- **crude data**—1. raw data. 2. unedited data. 3. **unadjusted data.**
- **data dredging**—Ad-hoc data analyses aimed at finding **statistically significant** differences among the different **subgroups** represented in a study, especially such analyses leading to a presentation heralding differences as being real and important. *Usage note*: Often used in a pejorative sense, especially in reference to analyses in which it appears that only large differences are presented and where the number of comparisons made is not specified.
- **dropout**—1. A person who withdraws from follow-up in a trial because of unwillingness to continue. 2. A person counted as a dropout because of an unbroken series of absences from scheduled followup visits. 3. One who refuses or stops taking the assigned treatment. *Usage note*: Most trials require continued data collection regardless of course of treatment if persons are willing. A dropout need not be **lost to follow-up** if investigators can determine outcome without seeing the person (e.g., as in some forms of follow-up for survival), but will be, if the outcome assessment depends on examination. Similarly, the act of dropping out need not affect **treatment compliance**. A person will become noncompliant upon dropping out when doing so results in discontinuation of an active treatment process. However, there may be no effect on treatment compliance in settings in which treatment is finished.
- **frequentist**—Being of or relating to a school of thought in which inferences depend on the probability distribution for parameter values based on the hypothetical notion of a study being repeated many times under the same conditions. See also: **Bayesian, likelihoodist.**
- **frequentist analysis**—A method of data analysis based on the notion that a study can be repeated many times under the same conditions and that inferences should be based on the hypothetical frequencies of repeated outcomes under a given hypothesis. Analyses are expressed as verdicts regarding the acceptance or

rejection of the **null hypothesis**; *p*-values are interpreted as an "observed" **type I error** rate or as represented in **confidence intervals**. *Usage note*: Most analyses in trials are of this form. Generally, the characterization "frequentist analysis" is used only in contradistinction to a method of analysis not requiring a frequentist view; e.g., as in **Bayesian analysis**.

- **intention-to-treat analysis**—Analysis by assigned treatment and one in which all persons assigned to treatment are counted to the assigned treatment group, regardless of course of treatment or of compliance to treatment.

- **interaction**—1. A relationship in which changes in response produced by treatments depend on other factors. 2. A relationship in which the nature or magnitude of the test-control **treatment difference** in a trial depends on one or more baseline characteristics. See also: **qualitative interaction, quantitative interaction**. *Usage note*: To be used as an explanation of an observed **treatment effect**, the variable in question should influence the size or nature of the treatment effect observed, and the difference should be large enough so as to be unlikely to be due to chance. Interaction and **confounding** have different conceptual bases and implications. In both cases, the variable in question must be related to outcome. In the case of confounding, the variable has to be differentially distributed by treatment group; in the case of interaction, the variable has to influence the **treatment difference** observed. The existence of an interaction does not affect one's ability to compare across treatment groups; the presence of a confounder does. Confounding influences one's certainty regarding the existence of a treatment effect since the difference can be explained by the treatments applied or by the confounding variable. Interaction influences one's certainty as to the extent to which a result applies across the spectrum of patients studied.

- **interacting variable**—1. In epidemiology, a variable that influences the size or nature of the effect observed (e.g., cigarette smoking in relation to lung cancer). 2. In trials, a variable that influences the nature or size of a **treatment difference**. See also: **confounding variable**.

Usage note: It is important, in the case of trials, to distinguish variables that are independent of treatment assignment (e.g., any variable observed before treatment assignment) from those that are not (any variable observed after the initiation of treatment). The distinction is important when trying to understand the biological relevance of the variable in the treatment process. An interaction effect due to a variable independent of treatment assignment; e.g., sex of the patients studied, is clearly of more importance in deciding how the treatment should be used, than for a variable not independent of treatment assignment.

- **interim look**—A mid-course look at trial results to determine whether the trial should be stopped or modified. See also: **multiple looks**.
- **interim result**—1. A result involving comparison of treatment groups during the trial. 2. Such a result leading to an **early stop**.
- **likelihoodist**—Being or relating to a school of thought for analysis and interpretation of data based on the **likelihood principle**. See also: **frequentist, Bayesian**.
- **likelihood principle**—A principle that asserts that all of the information for assessing evidence for one hypothesis versus an alternative hypothesis, given a set of data and an assumed model, is contained in the likelihood function of the hypotheses. In the case of trials, the principle implies that the interpretation of a dataset, in regard to the amount of support provided for one hypothesis versus another, is independent of the reason for the analysis; i.e., is not influenced by the number of **interim looks** performed in the past or by whether or not the trial was subject to a stopping rule.
- **lost to follow-up**—1. A person who cannot be found for **follow-up**. 2. A person unsuitable for follow-up because of some intervening condition or state. See also: **dropout**.
- **multiple comparisons**—1. Two or more comparisons involving the same measure; such comparison at the same point in time (as in the Coronary Drug Project,[30] involving comparison of pairs of treatments for a designated outcome at a single point in time); such comparison at different points in time (as in a particular

test-control treatment comparison for a particular outcome measure at different points in time). 2. Two or more comparisons involving different measures; such comparison at the same point in time; such comparisons at different points in time. 3. A comparison having an associated p-value or **confidence interval** that is adjusted to take account of the fact that it is one of several comparisons made. See also: **multiple looks**. *Usage note*: Virtually every trial involves multiple comparisons in the sense of definitions 1 and 2, even those involving just two study treatments. Any trial involving three or more study treatments and the need for two or more pairwise comparisons (as in the Coronary Drug Project, in the comparison of each of five different test treatments with a placebo control[30]) will involve multiple comparisons anytime the treatments are compared.

- **multiple looks**—Treatment comparisons made at two or more time points over the course of a trial; especially when done in relation to treatment effects monitoring and where they may lead to alteration of the treatment protocol. See also: **multiple comparisons**. *Usage note*: Not to be confused with **multiple comparisons**, as discussed in a usage note for that term.
- **null hypothesis**—1. A hypothesis that there is no difference in the populations or groups being compared with regard to a particular factor, trait, characteristic, condition, or treatment. See also: **alternative hypothesis**.
- **one-tailed alternative hypothesis**—A hypothesis serving as an alternative to the **null hypothesis** that specifies a range of permissible values of a parameter, all of which lie to one side of the null value (e.g., $H_o: \mu_1 = \mu_2$ versus $H_a: \mu_1 > \mu_2$). See also: **two-tailed alternative hypothesis**.
- p-**value**—Probability value associated with an observed **test statistic** that corresponds to the proportion of times one would expect to observe a value as extreme or more extreme than the one observed if the **null hypothesis** were true; e.g., a p-value of 0.05 for an observed result means that, on average, one in 20 replications of the study would be expected to yield a result as extreme or more extreme

than the one observed if the null hypothesis were true. *Usage note*: Traditionally, a p-value of 0.05 or smaller is taken as evidence of **statistical significance**. However, it is prudent to avoid that tradition, especially in settings in which the observed result and associated test statistic is just one among many of interest. It is better in that case to treat the p-values as additional descriptors of the observed data, rather than as quantitative indicators of statistical significance.

- **power**—The probability of rejecting the **null hypothesis** when it is false; one minus the **type II error**.

- **qualitative interaction**—An **interaction** in which the sign of the relationship for **subgroups** depends on the value assumed by the variable of interest; e.g., a treatment by gender interaction in which the treatment effect is positive for males and negative for females. See also: **quantitative interaction**.

- **quantitative interaction**—An **interaction** in which the sign of the **treatment difference** is the same for **subgroups** examined, but where the magnitude of the difference depends on the value assumed by the subgrouping variable; e.g., a treatment by gender interaction in which the treatment difference is larger for males than for females. See also: **qualitative interaction**.

- **sample size**—1. The number of sampling units to be drawn or selected for a sample; the number so selected or drawn. 2. The anticipated or actual number of elements or units constituting the database for a study; e.g., the number of patients to be enrolled into a trial or the number actually enrolled.

- **sample size calculation**—A mathematical calculation, usually carried out when a study is being planned, that indicates the number of observation or treatment units to be enrolled in order to provide a specified **type I** and **type II error** protection.

- **statistical significance**—1. p-**value** 2. An observed result that yields an appropriately small p-value (say, ≤ 0.05), using a specified **test of significance**.

- **statistically significant**—Marked by **statistical significance**.

- **subgroup**—A subset of a study population distinguished by a characteristic or set of characteristics; especially, in the case of trials, such a subset as distinguished by one or more baseline characteristics.

- **subgroup analysis**—A form of exploratory data analysis aimed at identifying a **subgroup** of persons that account for an observed difference; e.g., such an analysis in a trial to determine whether or not an observed **treatment difference** can be explained by some subgroup, especially such analysis using baseline characteristics for subgrouping. *Usage note*: Not to be confused with **data dredging**, which is a pejorative term. Subgroup analysis is neutral in connotation. Analysis involving subgroups formed using entry demographic and other baseline characteristics is an essential part of the analysis process for a trial. The analyses are done to determine whether it is reasonable to regard the treatment effect observed as being homogeneous (i.e., independent of entry and other important baseline characteristics). The analysis has bearing on conclusions reached from the trial. Evidence of **qualitative** or **quantitative interaction** obligates the trialist to temper or qualify conclusions accordingly. A **treatment effect** cannot be assumed to be homogeneous across subgroups absent analyses aimed at addressing questions of homogeneity of effect. Subgroup analyses become forms of data dredging if the results of such analyses are used to identify "significant" differences without regard to the number of subgroups studied or when the results are presented, so as to suggest that the difference reported is the result of clinical insight regarding an underlying disease process.
- **test of significance**—1. The evaluation of observed data by calculating a **test statistic** and using the result to decide whether to accept or reject the **null hypothesis**, as determined by whether the observed result lies in the acceptance or rejection region for the test. 2. The evaluation of observed data by calculating a specified test statistic and then deriving the *p*-**value** for the statistic.
- **test statistic**—1. The formula or computing algorithm used to carry out a **test of significance**. 2. The numerical value provided by the formula or computing algorithm for a specified test of significance using a defined dataset.

- **treatment compliance**—The degree to which a person or the person's treater follows the assigned treatment regimen.
- **treatment difference**—The signed difference of a subtraction of value for one treatment group versus another; typically, the test-assigned group versus the control-assigned group (e.g., the observed proportion dead in the test-assigned group versus the corresponding proportion in the control-assigned group).
- **treatment effect**—1. A quantity representing the change in response produced by a treatment, as in models for analysis of variance. 2. An effect attributed to the test treatment; in trials, usually inferred or estimated from a comparison of the test- and control-assigned groups. 3. The effect (adverse or beneficial) produced or assumed to be produced by a treatment in a person, usually assessed by measurements made before and after administration of the treatment. 4. **treatment difference**.
- **two-tailed alternative hypothesis**—A hypothesis serving as an alternative to the **null hypothesis** that specifies a range of permissible values of a parameter, symmetrically arrayed about the value (e.g., $H_0{:}\mu_1 = \mu_2$ versus $H_A{:}\mu_1 \; \mu_2$). See also: **one-tailed alternative hypothesis**.
- **type I error**—The probability of rejecting the **null hypothesis** when it is true, usually denoted by α. See also: **type II error**.
- **type II error**—The probability of accepting the **null hypothesis** when it is false, usually denoted by β. See also: **power, type I error**.
- **unadjusted data**—Data not subjected to **adjustment procedures**; raw data. *Usage note*: Data are assumed to be in their raw, unadjusted state unless otherwise specified.
- **uncontrolled**—Lacking a basis for comparison. *Usage note*: The term, in relation to trials and treatment assignments, is generally used to indicate the lack of an appropriate comparison or control group.

17

Subgroup Analysis vs. Data Dredging

There are three kinds of lies: Lies, damned lies and statistics.

Benjamin Disraeli

Suppose a single-center, randomized, double-masked trial is performed to assess the safety and efficacy of Drug X against a matching placebo for treatment of a life-limiting disease, that death is the primary outcome measure, and that the number of people enrolled is 200, evenly split between the two treatment groups.

The mortality results of the trial are presented in Table 17.1.

Overall, there is no mortality difference between the two treatment groups. The number of deaths in the two treatment groups was exactly the same, suggesting that Drug X was no better than a placebo in prolonging life. That being so, investigators would be justified in writing up their results and concluding that:

> We find no evidence to suggest that Drug X is any better than placebo in delaying deaths in our study population.

Table 17.1 Mortality results by treatment group

Drug X			Placebo			Comparison	
No. Rz*	Dead	%	No. Rz*	Dead	%	Diff†	p-value
100	25	25.0	100	25	25.0	0.0	1.00

* Number randomized.

† Diff = Difference in percent dead in Drug X assigned treatment group minus percent dead in placebo-assigned treatment group.

That would be the proper conclusion, provided the effect is homogeneous across the different types of patients represented in the trial—but trialists cannot be sure that is the case without checking. The usual way to do that is to look at treatment differences within subgroups of patients in the trial, defined by variables observed at or prior to the time of randomization (baseline data). (Variables observed after randomization are not suitable for such examination because their values may be influenced by treatment; hence "confounded" with treatment.)

But there are lots of possible subgroups that trialists could examine, even if they limit their examination to baseline variables. For example, suppose five binary baseline variables, such as having just two values, like male or female, or categorized into two mutually exclusive groups like persons on entry aged less than 60 or 60 or older. Those five variables would produce ten possible subgroups, two for each variable—thus, 240 possible subgroups, if variables are considered as pairs (e.g., as with the pair gender and age producing four possible subgroups; "possible" because some subgroups may be empty or so sparsely populated that it makes analysis meaningless).

Given the relatively small sample size in the trial, investigators are content to simply look for treatment differences in the six subgroups formed using gender, age, and race without any pairing. The results are presented in Table 17.2.

The table gives the breakdown of deaths by treatment group for the different subgroups and the number of people in the subgroups. The study

Table 17.2 Mortality results by gender, race, and age

Column no.	1	2	3	4	5	6	7	8
	Drug X			Placebo			Comparison	
	No. Rz*	Dead	%	No. Rz*	Dead	%	Diff†	p-value
Gender								
Males	50	19	38.0	50	12	24.0	14.0	0.19
Females	50	6	12.0	50	13	26.0	−14.0	0.12
Gender interaction							28.0	0.04
Race								
White	85	20	23.5	90	22	24.4	−0.9	1.00
Nonwhite	15	5	33.3	10	3	30.0	3.3	1.00
Skin color Interaction							2.4	0.04
Age at entry								
<60	20	2	10.0	15	3	20.0	−10.0	0.72
≥60	80	23	28.8	85	22	25.9	2.9	0.81
Age Interaction							−12.9	0.67

* Number randomized to treatment.

† Diff = Difference in percent dead in Drug X assigned treatment group minus percent dead in placebo-assigned treatment group.

population was evenly split between males and females, predominantly white, and aged 60 or older.

The values displayed in column 7 are differences in the percent dead in the drug-assigned group versus the percent dead in the placebo assigned group. The p-values (via the equivalent of Fisher's exact test) in column 8 require a little explanation. They represent the chance of observing a mortality difference equal to or more extreme than the one observed if the null hypothesis is true that the two treatments are the same in regard to prolonging life. For example, a p-value of 0.50 means that 50% of trials done under identical circumstances would yield a subgroup difference as large or larger than the one observed if, indeed, the two treatments are the same in regard to effect on mortality for that subgroup. P-values that are small, traditionally 0.05 or less, are taken as sufficient evidence to reject the null hypothesis (i.e., to regard it as not true). *Statistically significant* is the term used to refer to p-values that are small enough to allow one to reject the null hypothesis (usually p-values of ≤ 0.05) under ordinary testing circumstances.

The difference on the last line of each of the three panels is a difference of a difference—the treatment difference in one subgroup versus the difference in the complementary subgroup, an estimate of the interaction effect of the subgrouping variable on treatment.

Interaction effects may be qualitative or quantitative. A *qualitative interaction* is one in which the test treatment is beneficial in one subgroup and harmful in the other subgroup. A *quantitative interaction* is one in which the treatment effect for the test treatment is in the same direction in both subgroups, but is more pronounced in one of them.

Suppose you have duplicate universes with two sets of investigators having done the same trial and having produced the exact same results, with the only difference being that investigators in Universe A took the course *Clinical Trials 101* and those in Universe B took *Data Dredging 101* instead.

Investigators schooled in *Clinical Trials 101* are taught to focus on the main effect, as seen in Table 17.1, and to be skeptical of subgroup differences unless sizable. Investigators in Universe B are taught to scour results for subgroup differences and to regard a difference as real if it has a p-value 0.05 or less.

The gender difference catches the eye of both sets of investigators because there is a suggestion that the treatment is beneficial for females and harmful for males. But, not surprisingly, their conclusions are different.

Investigators in Universe A conclude:

> Results suggest Drug X is no better than placebo. There was no difference in mortality between the two treatment groups. The fraction dying was, in fact, the same: 25% in both treatment groups. We did subgroup analyses by

gender, skin color, and age as checks on homogeneity of treatment effects across subgroups. The only difference of note was for gender. The difference is suggestive of a gender-by-treatment interaction, but the difference may not be reproducible.

Investigators in Universe B conclude:

The results suggest that Drug X is beneficial in females and harmful in males. Only eight of the females enrolled died compared to 18 of the males assigned to Drug X. The p-value for a gender-by-treatment interaction was statistically significant ($p = 0.05$). The results raise questions as to whether the treatment should be used in males with the condition studied here. More research is needed to confirm the difference.

Both sets of investigators submit their papers for publication. Investigators in Universe A have to submit to four different journals before being published. The paper receives little notice. Investigators in Universe B hit pay-dirt on the first try. Their results make the evening news and newspapers around the country. It nets them interviews on CNN and CBS.

The results are the same. The only difference is how the investigators interpret them.

Suppose your father is taking Drug X, and he is happy taking it because of the pain relief it provides. Do you harass him and his doctor to have him come off the drug because of the chance of it shortening his life? You might, if you believe what Investigators in Universe B report. But is your concern justified? Probably not.

Why not?

First, because the trial is just one "flip of the coin" in the evaluation process of Drug X. It takes more than one trial to reveal "truth." You could go hunting for more trials, to try to gather more information to address your concern, but the chance of finding more is slim. You can be reasonably sure, if other trials exist supporting the conclusion of Investigators from Universe B, that they would have mentioned them in their paper.

Maybe, a decade or so later, after other trials on Drug X have been done, a meta-analysis or systematic review (Chapter 18) will provide reliable evidence on whether the treatment is good for females and bad for males—but that is years away.

The trial is relatively small and was done at a single center. You might have more faith that the treatment-by-gender effect is reproducible if the trial had been ten times larger and if the same gender difference was observed in most of the clinics in the trial.

Another reason to be suspicious is because the investigators made more of the p-value than they should. There is a price for scouring the data for "significant" differences, as implied by Cornfield[27] in picturesque terms:

> Just as the Sphinx winks if you look at it too long, so, if you perform enough significance tests you are sure to find significance, even when none exists.

The reason Investigators from Universe A downplayed the gender interaction effect was because they know that the chance of finding reproducible differences using conventional p-values of 0.05 to identify them will lead to a fair number of rejections of the null hypothesis when it is, in fact, true.

There is a price to be paid for multiple looks. The method for calculating the price is more than you need to know here. Suffice it to say that the p-value should be a lot smaller than 0.05 before investigators having taken Clinical Trials 101 get excited; perhaps as much as ten times smaller—0.005 instead of 0.05. Investigators in Universe B do not apply any "price." They just look for differences having a conventional p-value of 0.05 or less.

The reason why investigators in Universe A are cautious is because they know that most subgroup differences identified by subgroup analyses have a nasty habit of not reproducing in subsequent trials.[131] Subgroup analysis has earned a bad name because of investigators in Universe B. There is nothing wrong with subgroup analysis; indeed, one can argue that trialists are irresponsible if they do not do such analyses before drawing conclusions. As already noted, they need to know whether the effect observed is homogeneous across all individuals represented in the trial. They should not conclude that a treatment works across the spectrum of people studied if there is evidence that this is not so. They should make such examinations for important subgroups, whether or not planned when the trial was designed.

The trouble with subgroup analyses is, therefore, not in doing them, but rather in their interpretations. The fact that investigators do not report results of subgroup analyses does not mean that they were not done, as some would have you believe in regard to gender as a subgrouping variable. The belief that gender-by-treatment interactions are unrecognized because investigators do not look for them is usually false. Most journals have word and table limits. Authors are not likely to use their word and table budgets reporting subgroup analyses unless they think there is something to report. The best that can be expected is a sentence indicating that subgroup analyses were done for designated variables and that no differences were found.

18

Meta-analyses and Systematic Reviews

As we know, there are known knowns. There are things we know we know. We also know there are known unknowns. That is to say, we know there are some things we do not know. But there are also unknown unknowns, the ones we don't know we don't know.

Donald Rumsfeld

You go to your doctor and are told that your bone mineral density (BMD) is low. Your doctor suggests you take Fosamax once a week to combat the loss. That night, you see Sally Field on TV touting Boniva for the same condition, which needs to be taken only once a month. What to do?

Or, your husband, who has put on a few pounds in recent years, goes for his annual checkup and his doctor tells him that his blood sugar is high and requests that he come back for a glucose tolerance test. The results suggest he has type 2 diabetes. His doctor gives him the usual spiel about diet and exercise and indicates he can likely control his blood sugar by diet and exercise alone. He comes home a changed man, compulsive about sticking to his new diet and newfound exercise routine—for awhile. Eventually, his blood sugar is back where it was before he started on his diet and exercise routine; his doctor suggests an oral antidiabetic agent to control his blood sugar, specifically Avandia. What to do?

You can, of course, go to PubMed or PubMed Central to find individual trials relevant to these questions, but which ones? And what will you make of the results when finished with that exercise?

The better, more efficient, approach is to look for meta-analyses or systematic reviews germane to your questions. Broadly, a **meta-analysis** (a term coined by Gene Glass in 1976[53]) is an analysis using either aggregate results or individual patient data from published trials. It is done to provide a more comprehensive and informative view of results than is possible with any single trial.

Meta-analysis, as a publication type (ptyp), was introduced by the National Library of Medicine, in 1993 and is defined as:

> Works consisting of studies using a quantitative method of combining the results of independent studies (usually drawn from the published literature) and synthesizing summaries and conclusions which may be used to evaluate therapeutic effectiveness, plan new studies, etc. It is often an overview of clinical trials. It is usually called a meta-analysis by the author or sponsoring body and should be differentiated from reviews of literature.

There were 2,463 publications in 2007 indexed to that publication type (limited to English and human-subject studies) and 17,672 regardless of year of publication (as of November 24, 2008).

A related activity is **systematic review** (aka *overview*). Such reviews, as applied to trials, typically involve efforts to identify all trials relevant to the question of interest, whether published or not, critical appraisals of the trials, and ultimately, a conclusion as to the weight of evidence for or against the treatment. Such reviews may or may not involve formal meta-analyses. Most meta-analyses, in contrast with systematic reviews, are based exclusively on published trials. The best place to find systematic reviews is in the Cochrane Library. It contains several thousand systematic reviews with new ones added regularly (http://mrw.interscience.wiley.com/cochrane/cochrane_clsysrev_articles_fs.html).

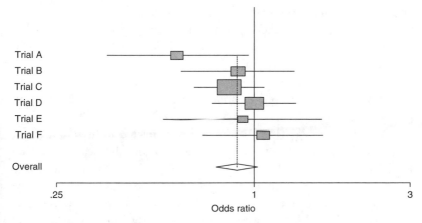

Figure 18.1 Forest plot.

A difficulty in all meta-analyses and systematic reviews is the identification of trials for inclusion. Obviously, it is imperative that the decisions be independent of trial results if the analysis or review is to be unbiased.

The issue of identification and selection is illustrated in the reports from the Antithrombotic Trialists' Collaboration, as cited in Chapter 19. In their 2002 publication,[8] investigators reported identifying 448 of them, but ended up rejecting 166 of the trials: 52 were not properly randomized, 24 were "confounded" (involved designs including non-antiplatelet treatments), 3 had large numbers lost to follow-up, 13 were abandoned or stopped before investigators had collected any outcome data, 20 had a cross-over design, and 54 did not have data for relevant outcome measures.

The usual way results are presented when based on aggregating results from individual trials is by use of *forest plots*,[73] as shown in Figure 18.1, for a hypothetical situation involving six trials.

The plots involve lines corresponding to trials and in which lengths correspond to 95% confidence intervals of the observed treatment differences. The lines are superimposed on a grid of lines corresponding to relative risk or odds. Lines to the right of the 1.0 vertical line (the line of no difference between the treatment groups) show trials in which the differences favor the study treatment. Lines to the left correspond to trials favoring the comparison treatment. Lines crossing the line correspond to trials not showing a significant treatment effect. The ordering of studies represented in the plots is usually in ascending order by time (e.g., as in the publication by Antman et al.).[10]

Now, back to the first question posed at the start of this chapter: Fosamax (alendronate) versus Boniva (ibandronate), or nothing at all for bone loss?

You start by searching for meta-analyses related to these questions. Entering "meta-analysis[ptyp] AND fractures" in the search field in PubMed produces 69 hits (search limited to 2007 or beyond; done November 27, 2008). Among the hits, papers titled "Systematic Review: Comparative Effectiveness of Treatments to Prevent Fractures in Men and Women with Low Bone Density or Osteoporosis" by MacLean et al.[75] and "Alendronate for the Primary and Secondary Prevention of Osteoporotic Fractures in Postmenopausal Women" by Wells et al.[129] are relevant.

The editors of the journal (*Annals of Internal Medicine*) publishing the MacLean et al. results state:

> This systematic review of 76 randomized trials and 24 meta-analyses found good evidence that multiple agents, including alendronate, zoledronic acid, and estrogen, prevented vertebral and hip fractures more than placebo. Harms included increased risk for thromboembolic events with raloxifene, estrogen, and estrogen-progestin, and increased gastrointestinal symptoms with bisphosphonates. No large trials directly compared two or more agents and established superiority of any agent.

But they caution that:

> Available data insufficiently characterize the benefits and harms of various therapies for osteoporosis relative to one another.

Wells and coworkers report a meta-analysis of 11 randomized alendronate trials representing 12,068 women. They conclude:

> At 10 mg per day, both clinically important and statistically significant reductions in vertebral, non-vertebral, hip and wrist fractures were observed for secondary prevention. We found no statistically significant results for

primary prevention, with the exception of vertebral fractures, for which the reduction was clinically important.

Note: The 10 mg per day dose corresponds to a weekly dose of 70 mg of Fosamax—the standard dose for that drug.)

As to comparison of the 70 mg weekly dose of Fosamax versus the 150 mg once-monthly dose of Boniva, only one trial provides a head-to-head comparison of the two drugs—a multicenter randomized, double-blind, noninferiority trial.[85] The authors conclude:

> Once-monthly ibandronate was shown to be clinically comparable to weekly alendronate at increasing BMD after 12 months in both the lumbar spine and total hip.[85]

The results from Wells et al. indicate the case for treatment is strongest for people with a history of fractures, a factor you need to consider when making your decision. What is your history?

As to Fosamax versus Boniva: There is not much to guide you. Obviously, the convenience of once-a-month versus once-a-week dosing is a consideration, but safety is more important. In this regard, the likelihood is that the two drugs are about the same. The label inserts for both drugs contain similar warnings, including warnings of a rare and disfiguring jaw condition—osteonecrosis of the jaw (ONJ). The condition in users of Fosamax has led to lawsuits against its manufacturer. But Fosamax has been in use longer than Boniva; Fosamax was approved in the fall of 1995 and Boniva, for once-monthly use, in the spring of 2005. The absence of similar claims against Boniva does not mean they will not emerge as use increases.

Next, let's consider whether your husband should take Avandia for his high blood sugar. Before deciding on whether to take the drug, your husband needs to know that drugs approved for use as blood sugar–lowering agents in type 2 diabetics are approved for use if they are shown to be safe and effective in lowering blood sugar levels. There are still questions among medical experts as to whether such control confers benefits in reduced risks of morbidity and mortality. The presumption is that it does, but it is a largely untested presumption.

If he is ready to accept the presumption, he is ready for the question of whether to go on Avandia. As with the bone loss question, you go to PubMed and enter "meta-analysis[ptyp] AND Avandia" and get 22 hits (November 28, 2008). You look through the list and settle on a paper by Nissen and Wolski entitled "Effect of Rosiglitazone on the Risk of Myocardial Infarction and Death from Cardiovascular Causes."[98] To make certain that rosiglitazone is just another name for Avandia you Google "Avandia" and go to Wikipedia (http://en.wikipedia.org/wiki/Rosiglitazone), which indicates that:

> Rosiglitazone is an anti-diabetic drug in the thiazolidinedione class of drugs. It is marketed by the pharmaceutical company GlaxoSmithKline as a stand-alone drug (Avandia) and in combination with metformin (Avandamet) or with glimepiride (Avandaryl). Annual sales approx $2.5bn [billion]. Patent expires 2012.

The paper indicates that the authors have combined data from 42 randomized trials that, together, include 15,500 patients assigned to receive rosiglitazone alone or in combination with other antidiabetic agents, and 12,290 patients assigned to control treatments of placebo or other blood sugar lowering agents.

Their conclusion:

> Rosiglitazone was associated with a significant increase in the risk of myocardial infarction and with an increase in the risk of death from cardio-vascular causes that had borderline significance. Our study was limited by a lack of access to original source data, which would have enabled time-to-event analysis. Despite these limitations, patients and providers should consider the potential for serious adverse cardiovascular effects of treatment with rosiglitazone for type 2 diabetes.

Alas, this is another judgment call as to whether the benefits of control via a drug like Avandia outweigh the potential risks.

19

Re-Search

New opinions often appear first as jokes and fancies, then as blasphemies and treason, then as questions open to discussion, and finally as established truths.

George Bernard Shaw

My wife is the family physician, Susan J. Meinert, WMD (Without Medical Degree). She is the one up to speed on the latest results from trials. She is constantly reminding me of things I should know. When she hears of new results on TV that contradict earlier results, she pokes at air, turns to no one in particular, and asks, "Why can't they make up their mind?"

I could, of course, remind her that there is no "they" when it comes to research, but you do not have to be married for very many years before you learn that silence is the best policy. So, I sit silent, biting my tongue, because if I were to say anything it would most likely come across like my chemistry professor puffing himself up to respond to some student. Only I would say in my own best high-pitched voice, "Well, the name of the game is *re*-search" with an elongated "re" and a two-second pause before mouthing the word "search," and then go back to my own scribbling. But I (usually) don't!

The fact is that truth in medicine is elusive and fleeting. That which is "truth" today is passé tomorrow. In regard to the way truth triumphs, it is, in large measure, as Max Planck (1858–1947), the renowned German physicist, said:

> A new scientific truth does not triumph by convincing its opponents and making them see the light, but rather because its opponents eventually die, and a new generation grows up that is familiar with it.*

When Ambroise Paré (1510–1590; French surgeon) was on the field during the battle to capture the castle of Villaine (1537), the standard treatment for gunshot wounds consisted of pouring boiling oil over the wound. When Paré ran out of oil during the battle he resorted to a digestive medicament made of egg yolks, oil of roses, and turpentine. The next day Paré wrote:

> I raised myself very early to visit them, when beyond my hope I found those to whom I had applied the digestive medicament feeling but little pain, their wounds neither swollen nor inflamed, and having slept through the night. The others to whom I had applied the boiling oil were feverish, with much pain and swelling about their wounds. Then I determined never again to burn thus so cruelly the poor wounded by arquebuses.[102]

But the practice of inflicting trauma to treat wounds persisted well after Paré. Pruitt, Pruitt, and Davis, in the opening chapter of a book entitled *Trauma* wrote:

> Like most steps forward, this [rejection of cautery] was by no means accepted by the majority of surgeons, and the idea that suppuration was a sign of good wound healing continued until the 20th century.[107]

George Washington's hypertension was treated with bloodletting and leeches. The practice faded from use in favor of potions, tonics, elixirs, and electricity, and eventually gave way to the use of drugs in the 1950s.[52]

---

* Translation from *Wissenschaftliche Selbstbiographie. Mit einem Bildnis und der von Max von Laue gehaltenen Traueransprache* (Leipzig 1948). Scientific Autobiography and Other Papers, trans F Gaynor (New York, 1949), pp 33–34 (as cited in TS Kuhn, *The Structure of Scientific Revolutions*).

When I relate stories such as these to students, I see flickers of disbelief. Those flickers cause me to remind them that there will be somebody like me standing in front of their progeny 200 years hence reciting similar stories—the only difference being that the stories will be about treatments in vogue today!

The tried-and-true method of coming to what we accept as "truth" in science is by replication. Remember the hoopla in the spring of 1989 surrounding a press conference at the University of Utah, when Stanley Pons and Martin Fleischmann announced that they had perfected cold fusion? The announcement was greeted with excitement and worldwide press coverage. But there was just one problem—no one was able to replicate their findings following the announcement.

For the most part, findings in the laboratory and clinical sciences are not taken as "proven" until they are replicated by others. Indeed, one of the purposes underlying publication in those sciences is to provide templates for replication. But the proof deriving from replication is different in the two sciences. In regard to the laboratory sciences and cold fusion, we might well be on our way to energy independence if anyone, anywhere in the world, had been able to replicate the work of Pons and Fleischmann.

Replication, in the strict sense of usage, is impossible in trials. No two trials are the same. The enrollment criteria will differ, the data collection schedules will differ, the treatment protocols will differ, even the treatments may be different. Hence, a single trial that reproduces a positive result seen in a previous trial is not sufficient to establish the value of that treatment. It takes multiple trials, usually spanning a period of years if not decades.

Truth emerges slowly and in an unsteady fashion, as noted by my wife every time she pokes at the air.

There is no "trial master" in the sky. There is nobody to ensure a stream of trials until a consensus view develops. Nor is there anyone to shut off trials once the "answer is in." Replication becomes duplication when the answer is in. But, when is that point reached? There is no bright line of demarcation.

Savulescu and coworkers[113] argue that institutional review boards/ ethics committees should require systematic reviews and meta-analyses of investigators proposing trials; in effect, to allow IRBs/ethics committees to decide whether the trials proposed are justified. But such efforts are major undertakings in their own right and, alone, can take years to complete.

Cumulative meta-analyses (a meta-analysis in which trials are ordered by the time in which results are combined, one trial at a time, to yield point and interval estimates of effect size as trials are added) have been used to highlight cases in which trials have been replicated to the point of duplication (e.g., as in Fergusson et al.).[41]

But, for every case in which people would say, "enough already," there are many more in which no or very little replication occurs. Indeed, the concern, as a society, should be more about the lack of replication of trials than with worries of investigators crossing the line of demarcation separating replication from duplication.

By and large, the bigger the trial, the less likely it is to be replicated and, hence, the more likely it is to be accepted as "truth." For example, it is unlikely that the Women's Health Initiative (WHI) primary prevention trial in postmenopausal women comparing estrogen plus progestin versus placebo will be replicated. One can argue that it should be because, after all, it is but one "flip of the coin." To be sure, one big and costly coin flip, but nonetheless just one flip. The fact that it is multicenter and that the negative effect reproduced across clinics gives added faith as to the "truth" of the result—but big is not synonymous with truth.

An added problem in replicating trials producing negative effects (as opposed to nil or positive effects) is the ethics of replication. Trials are done in the hope of showing positive effects, not to establish ill effects.

The ability to do trials depends on money to fund them and on a cadre of investigators willing to undertake them. Willingness depends on the perceived importance of the information that will be generated, on whether the trial is feasible, and on whether it is justifiable on ethical grounds. Investigators and IRBs alike will be reluctant to proceed if a state of clinical equipoise is perceived to no longer exist (see Chapter 8).

The ethical underpinning of trials depends on the prevailing view of "truth." If results from a previous trial suggest that a treatment is harmful, there may not be investigators willing to undertake another trial for fear of finding the same thing. For example, there is no doubt that the adverse mortality results for the oral agents tested in the University Group Diabetes

Program (UGDP)[125,126] limited the options for follow-on studies and the willingness of others to undertake replications of the trial.

The same is true for positive results, especially in relation to serious life-threatening or life-limiting diseases. There is a tendency to take such results as "established," without further testing. A case in point is AIDS Clinical Trials Group (ACTG) Protocol 079. The protocol produced positive results suggesting that zidovudine was effective in interdicting vertical transmission of HIV from mothers to newborns.[76] *

Following those results, investigators in Thailand and Uganda did trials to see if lesser regimens of drugs would also interdict transmission. Although their results were encouraging, they and their sponsors were roundly criticized by those who regarded the dosage and treatment schedules used there to be suboptimum, as measured against dosages and schedules used in ACTG Protocol 079 (see also Chapter 11).

By and large, large-scale multicenter trials are not done to assess safety. A notable exception is the Prospective Randomized Evaluation of Celecoxib Integrated Safety vs. Ibuprofen or Naproxen (PRECISION) trial. The trial, still ongoing, is sponsored by Pfizer and estimated to cost $100 million when completed.[31] It came about as a result of widespread concerns that the class of nonsteroidal anti-inflammatory drugs (NSAIDs) used for pain relief in arthritis carried cardiovascular risks for users. The trial is designed to determine the relative safety of celecoxib (Celebrex), ibuprofen (Motrin), and naproxen (Naprosyn or Aleve).

The most fertile setting for "replication" is in the presence of nil results trending toward positive. A case in point is the spate of trials done to assess the usefulness of aspirin or other antiplatelet drugs for prevention of vascular events.

Randomized, controlled trials involving aspirin to assess its value in preventing vascular events started to come to publication in the 1970s.

---

* The trial produced a 67.5% relative reduction in HIV transmission, corresponding to a p-value of 0.00006 and widely regarded as providing definitive proof of the benefit of treatment. As trials go, the one done under Protocol 079 is relatively small, involving 383 mothers delivering newborns during the trial, with 180 women assigned to receive zidovudine and 183 women assigned to receive a matching placebo.

Those early trials were done to assess the usefulness of the drug in preventing myocardial infarctions (MIs) by people having a history of MI. Canner looked at the first six of these trials in a 1983 publication.[21]

Five of the trials produced results suggestive of benefit for aspirin and one, the largest of the six trials ($n = 2,267$), produced results suggesting that aspirin was inferior to the control treatment (placebo). None of the differences in any of the trials were statistically significant.

Now fast forward to 1994. In that year, the Antithrombotic Trialists' Collaboration published a meta-analysis of 145 randomized trials of antiplatelet therapy involving people with a history of vascular disease or at high risk of presenting with vascular disease.[9] By 2002, and their second such meta-analysis, they had an additional 52 trials,[8] and the number of people represented in the analysis had grown from 70,000 to 135,000.

Their conclusion was that:

> Aspirin (or another oral antiplatelet drug) is protective in most types of patients at increased risk of occlusive vascular events, including those with an acute myocardial infarction or ischemic stroke, unstable or stable angina, previous myocardial infarction, stroke or cerebral ischemia, peripheral arterial disease, or atrial fibrillation.[8]

This accumulation of data led to the widespread daily use of "baby aspirin" in people having a history of vascular events or considered to be at high risk of vascular events.

So, what about aspirin or other antiplatelet drugs for primary prevention of coronary heart disease? Utilizing six randomized trials published over a span of 16 years (1988–2005), representing 47,000 participants, Bartolucci and Howard[13] concluded:

> [P]rimary prevention with aspirin decreased the risk of total CHD, nonfatal MI, and total CV events, but there were no significant differences in the incidence of stroke or CV mortality.

Individually, only two of the trials yielded statistically significant results favoring aspirin. The other four had 95% confidence intervals overlapping the zero point of no difference.

A few years earlier (2002), the U.S. Preventive Services Task Force (USPSTF) based its conclusion on five of the six trials analyzed by Bartolucci and Howard:

The USPSTF found good evidence that aspirin decreases the incidence of coronary heart disease in adults who are at increased risk for heart disease. It also found good evidence that aspirin increases the incidence of gastrointestinal bleeding and fair evidence that aspirin increases the incidence of hemorrhagic strokes. The USPSTF concluded that the balance of benefits and harms is most favorable in patients at high risk for coronary heart disease (those with a 5-year risk ≥3%) but is also influenced by patient preferences.[127]

A meta-analysis of the same six trials to look for sex differences in response to treatment was done by Berger et al.[16] in 2006. Their conclusion was that:

For women and men, aspirin therapy reduced the risk of a composite of cardiovascular events due to its effect on reducing the risk of ischemic stroke in women and MI in men. Aspirin significantly increased the risk of bleeding to a similar degree among women and men.

Ogawa et al., for the Japanese Primary Prevention of Atherosclerosis with Aspirin for Diabetes (JPAD),[101] in a multicenter randomized trial involving 2,539 type 2 diabetics, concluded that:

[L]ow-dose aspirin as primary prevention did not reduce the risk of cardiovascular events

but, in reality, the results are consistent with benefit for aspirin, albeit, not with differences large enough to produce statistical significance (p-values ≤0.05). Their summary of results, as given in the abstract of their paper, is as follows:

A total of 154 atherosclerotic events occurred: 68 in the aspirin group (13.6 per 1000 person-years) and 86 in the nonaspirin group (17.0 per 1000 person-years) (hazard ratio [HR], 0.80; 95% confidence interval [CI], 0.58–1.10; log-rank test, P = .16). The combined endpoint of fatal coronary events and fatal cerebrovascular events occurred in 1 patient (stroke) in the aspirin group and 10 patients (5 fatal myocardial infarctions and 5 fatal strokes) in the non-aspirin group (HR, 0.10; 95% CI, 0.01–0.79; $P = .0037$). A total of 34 patients in the aspirin group and 38 patients in the nonaspirin group died from any cause (HR, 0.90; 95% CI, 0.57–1.14; log-rank test, $P = .67$). The composite of hemorrhagic stroke and significant gastrointestinal bleeding was not significantly different between the aspirin and nonaspirin groups.

So, where do things stand?

The consensus is that the benefits deriving from daily use of aspirin and similar type drugs outweigh the possible ill-effects in secondary prevention of vascular disease.

Where are we in pursuit of "truth" in regard to primary prevention? That "truth" is still emerging.

And those, my dear, are some of the reasons why "They can't make up their mind!"

20

Shopping for a Trial?

For true success ask yourself these four questions: Why? Why not? Why not me? Why not now?

James Allen

Suppose you or one of yours has just been diagnosed with a serious condition for which there is no established treatment. Would you shop for a trial to join? Alternatively, suppose your doctor tells you of a randomized trial involving tests of relevance to you. Would you enroll in it?

Consider first the shopping question.

If you listen to the radio or read local newspapers, you will hear or see ads for trials, but they are unlikely to be of relevance to your particular situation. As a rule, they relate to efforts to recruit for a prevention trial, or more likely, phase II or III short-term trials; those sponsored by drug companies in relation to new drug applications.

In general, if in such ads there is an offer of pay for joining or per completed visit, you can be reasonably certain the trial is not relevant. You are looking for a treatment trial and, as a rule, there is no offer of pay in such trials (as discussed in Chapter 8). The likelihood of the offer of pay diminishes with the seriousness of the condition being treated and with the prospect of direct benefit from the trial.

By and large, you should be shopping for randomized trials. You may be willing to be among the first persons exposed to a new treatment, absent any control treatment or randomization (e.g., with a possible gene therapy treatment), but the risk–benefit calculus in that setting is different from that in randomized trials. With randomized trials you can be reasonably certain of two things:

1. That there was a series of trials prior to the one of interest showing the treatment to be reasonably safe, and
2. That there is an underlying state of clinical equipoise (discussed in Chapter 8).

A question you will have to face is whether you are willing to accept any of the treatments being tested. If the control treatment is a placebo, you have to decide whether you would be willing to receive it. If the answer is no, there may not be any trials to shop for.

So, how do you shop for a trial?

You Google of course. Start with *clinicaltrials.gov*. The site is a registry of 97,000+ trials (as of October 14, 2010) in different stages, ranging from still being planned to completed, and everything in between. Chances are that you will find some trials relevant to you and that they are open for enrollment.

Enter the condition diagnosed. The website gives information on where the trials are being done, whether they are open for enrollment, who sponsors them, general eligibility criteria, and contact information.

Other registration sites include:

- http://www.anzctr.org.au (Australian New Zealand Clinical Trials Registry)
- http://www.isrctn.org (International Standard Randomised Controlled Trial Number Register)
- http://www.trialregister.nl/trialreg/index.asp (Netherlands Trial Registry)

- http://www.umin.ac.jp/ctr (Japan University Hospital Medical Information Network Clinical Trials Registry).

You can also surf the web for ongoing trials listed on the websites of major drug companies.

So, OK, however it happens, suppose you are presented with the prospect of enrolling in a randomized trial. What are the deciding factors? Decisions are highly personal, so there is no generic formula, but there are indicators that can guide you. One guide, developed specifically for this book, is presented in Appendix C: A Patient's Guide for Deciding Whether to Enroll in a Randomized Trial. A suitable match for you is one in which all the questions are answered "yes." Any "no" answer should give you pause as to joining. (Note that the guide is for consideration of enrollment into a randomized controlled trial. Obviously, the questions would be different if the trial is not randomized, as is typically the case with phase I or II trials.)

Ideally, the people who designed the trial you are considering can answer all the questions in "The Mother Test" (see Appendix A) in the affirmative. If you doubt that to be the case, you should not enroll.

You should be suspicious of any trial in which you are "rushed" to make a decision. Your responsibility is to understand what will be involved before signing on. No good is served by rushing. If you are uncertain whether you will be able to stick with the trial, do yourself and the study a favor: decline enrollment.

You have the right to withdraw at any time after enrollment, without prejudice, but you should not enroll if "withdrawal" is your "bailout" if you do not like the treatment assignment. Trials are degraded by dropouts and losses to follow-up. Losses can render an otherwise good trial largely worthless.

You can withdraw from the trial, but you can't withdraw the data that has been collected on you. You need to understand that before you enroll. Allowing withdrawal of data opens the results of the entire trial to debilitating biases.

Except for trials done in emergency settings, you should expect to be given a copy of the consent form and ample time to read it and to consider your decision before being asked to sign it. In general, being presented with a consent form and being asked to sign on the spot is an indicator of a staff more concerned with the form of consent than with its substance. The consenting process varies depending on the age and ability of persons to consent. Adults (those aged 18 and older), have power of consent except if not mentally competent to make informed judgments. Sometimes the power extends to persons less than 18 in cases of research involving emancipated minors (e.g., as in some teenage pregnancy studies).

IRBs vary as to "age of assent"—the age at which the assent of the child is required in order to be studied; usually this is the age of 6 but IRBs vary some as to age. The parent or child's guardian has to consent and the child has to assent in order to study the child.

The consenting process for adults who are mentally incompetent involves something roughly akin to assent of the person to be studied and consent of the person's guardian or surrogate.

If specimens are banked, the consent form should indicate that fact, who has access to specimens, and whether results of tests done on specimens will be made known to you.

Institutional review boards want consents that inform people exactly how long they can be expected to be followed and when the study will end, but that is not always possible. Hence, you may expect some imprecision in that regard. You should not enroll if the imprecision makes you uneasy.

If you are not willing to accept whatever treatment is assigned by the randomization process, you should not enroll.

Some consents may include mention of the fact that, because it is important to keep track of everybody, at least in regard to whether alive or dead, efforts will be made to determine whether persons are still living or dead, even if they drop out. Such tracking methods are typically done by resorting to agencies expert in making such determinations without direct contact with the persons enrolled. You should not enroll if that makes you uncomfortable.

21

Readings

I don't think much of a man who is not wiser today than he was yesterday.

Abraham Lincoln

If you made it this far, you should know a little bit more than when you started. You may not be ready to go out and design a trial, but you know something about how they are put together, what makes them tick, and even a little bit about what to make of their results. So how about a reading list of references to further your education?

Textbooks

Every trialist needs a library of standard textbooks. Clearly, it should include texts on the nuts and bolts of trials, texts on biostatistics, and texts devoted to the ethics of medical research.

Biostatistics

Altman, Douglas G. 1991. *Practical Statistics for Medical Research.* London: Chapman & Hall. 16 chapters, 2 appendices, 611 pp.

Chow, Shein-Chung; Shao, Jun; Wang, Hanshang. 2003. *Sample Size Calculations in Clinical Research*. New York: Marcel Dekker. 12 chapters, 1 appendix, 372 pp.

Diggle, Peter J.; Heagerty, Patrick J.; Liang, Kung-Yee; Zeger, Scott L. 2002. *Analysis of Longitudinal Data*. New York: Oxford University Press. 14 chapters, 6 appendices, 379 pp.

Donner, Allan; Klar, Neil. 2000. *Design and Analysis of Cluster Randomization Trials in Health Research*. New York: Oxford University Press. 9 chapters; 178 pp.

Hill, Austin Bradford. 1955. *Principles of Medical Statistics*, 6th edition. New York: Oxford University Press, 1955. 314 pp.

Hill, Austin Bradford. 1962. *Statistical Methods in Clinical and Preventive Medicine*. New York: Oxford University Press. 610 pp.

Jennison, Christopher; Turnbull, Bruce W. 1999. *Group Sequential Methods with Applications to Clinical Trials*. London: Chapman & Hall. 19 chapters, 390 pp.

Petitti, Diana B. 2000. *Meta-analysis, Decision Analysis and Cost-effectiveness Analysis: Methods for Quantitative Synthesis in Medicine*, 2nd edition. New York: Oxford University Press. 17 chapters, 306 pp.

Shuster, Jonathan. 1990. *CRC Handbook of Sample Size Guidelines for Clinical Trials*. Boca Raton, FL: CRC Press. 3 chapters, 2 appendices, 854 pp.

van Belle, Gerald; Fisher, Lloyd D.; Heagerty, Patrick J.; Lumley, Thomas S. 2004.*Biostatistics: A Methodology for the Health Sciences*, 2nd edition. New York: John Wiley & Sons. 20 chapters, 1 appendix, 896 pp.

Clinical Trials

Armitage, Peter. 1975. *Sequential Medical Trials*, 2nd edition. New York: John Wiley & Sons. 194 pp.

Berger, Vance W. 2005. *Selection Bias and Covariate Imbalances in Randomized Clinical Trials*. New York: John Wiley & Sons. 8 chapters, 218 pp.

Buyse, Marc E.; Staquet, Maurice J.; Sylvester, Richard J. 1984. *Cancer Clinical Trials: Methods and Practice*. New York: Oxford University Press. 25 chapters, 481 pp.

Chow, Shein-Chung; Liu, Jen-Pei. 2003. *Design and Analysis of Clinical Trials: Concepts and Methodologies*, 2nd edition. New York: John Wiley & Sons. 15 chapters; 752 pp.

Ellenberg, Susan S.; Fleming, Thomas R.; DeMets, David L. 2002. *Data Monitoring Committees in Clinical Trials: A Practical Perspective*. New York: John Wiley & Sons. 10 chapters, 1 appendix, 191 pp.

Fleiss, Joseph L. 1986. *Design and Analysis of Clinical Experiments*. New York: John Wiley & Sons. 13 chapters, 1 appendix, 432 pp.

Friedman, Lawrence M.; Furberg, Curt D.; DeMets David L. 1998. *Fundamentals of Clinical Trials*, 3rd edition. New York: Springer. 19 chapters, 361 pp.

Hayes, Richard J.; Moulton, Lawrence H. 2009. *Cluster Randomized Trials: A Practical Approach*. Boca Raton, FL: Chapman & Hall/CRC Press. 338 pp.

Herson, Jay. 2009. *Data and Safety Monitoring Committees in Clinical Trials*. Boca Raton, FL: Chapman & Hall/CRC. 173 pp.

Meinert, Curtis L.; Tonascia, Susan. 1986. *Clinical Trials: Design, Conduct, and Analysis*. New York: Oxford University Press. 26 chapters, 9 appendices, 469 pp.

Piantadosi, Steven. 2005. *Clinical Trials: A Methodologic Perspective*, 2nd edition. New York: John Wiley & Sons. 22 chapters, 8 appendices, 687 pp.

Rosenberger, William F.; Lachin, John M. 2002. *Randomization in Clinical Trials: Theory and Practice*. New York: John Wiley & Sons. 15 chapters, 258 pp.

Senn, Stephen. 2002. *Cross-over Trials in Clinical Research*. New York: John Wiley & Sons. 10 chapters, 345 pp.

Smith, Peter G.; Morrow, Richard H. 1996. *Field Trials of Health Interventions in Developing Countries: A Toolbox*, 2nd edition. New York: Macmillian. 16 chapters, 362 pp.

Whitehead, John. 1997. *The Design and Analysis of Sequential Clinical Trials*, 2nd edition. New York: John Wiley & Sons. 9 chapters, 1 appendix, 328 pp.

Ethics

Beauchamp, Tom L.; Faden, Ruth R.; Wallace, R.J. Jr.; Walters, L. 1982. *Ethical Issues in Social Science Research*. Baltimore: The Johns Hopkins University Press 19 chapters, 436 pp.

Faden, Ruth R.; Beauchamp, Tom L.; King, Nancy M. P. 1986. *A History and Theory of Informed Consent*. New York: Oxford University Press. 10 chapters; 392 pp.

Levine, Robert J. 1988. *Ethics and Regulation of Clinical Research*, 2nd edition. New Haven, CT: Yale University Press. 14 chapters, 5 appendices, 452 pp.

Silverman, William A. 1985. *Human Experimentation: A Guided Step into the Unknown*. New York: Oxford University Press. 12 chapters, 2 appendices, 204 pp.

History

Marks, Harry M. 1997. *The Progress of Experiment: Science and Therapeutic Reform in the United Sates, 1900–1990*. Cambridge: Cambridge University Press. 8 chapters; 258 pp.

Clinical Research

Kolman, Josef; Meng, Paul; Scott, Graeme, eds. 1998. *Good Clinical Practice: Standard Operating Procedures for Clinical Researchers.* New York: John Wiley & Sons. 210 pp.

Data Management

McFadden, Eleanor. 1998. *Management of Data in Clinical Trials.* New York: John Wiley & Sons. 12 chapters, 210 pp.

Meta-analysis

Egger, Matthias; Smith, George Davey; Altman, Douglas G., eds. 2001. *Systematic Reviews in Health Care: Meta-analysis in Context.* London: BMJ Publishing Group. 26 chapters, 487 pp.

Glasziou, Paul; Irwig, Les; Bain, Chris; Colditz, Graham. 2001. *Systematic Reviews in Health Care: A Practical Guide.* Cambridge: Cambridge University Press. 10 chapters, 2 appendices, 137 pp.

Whitehead, Annie. 2002. *Meta-analysis of Controlled Clinical Trials.* New York: John Wiley & Sons. 12 chapters, 1 appendix, 352 pp.

Epidemiology

Hulley, Stephen B.; Cummings, Steven R.; Browner, Warren S.; Grady, Deborah; Hearst, Norman; Newman, Thomas B. 2001. *Designing Clinical Research: An Epidemiological Approach*, 2nd edition. Philadelphia: Lippincott Williams & Wilkins. 19 chapters, 336 pp.

Statistics

Salsburg, David. 2001. *The Lady Tasting Tea: How Statistics Revolutionized Science in the Twentieth Century.* New York: WH Freeman. 29 chapters, 352 pp.

Public Health

Brownson, Ross C.; Baker, Elizabeth A.; Leet, Terry L.; Gillespie, Kathleen N. 2003. *Evidence-Based Public Health.* New York: Oxford University Press. 9 chapters, 235 pp.

General Guide

Woodin, Karen E. 2004. *The CRC's Guide to Coordinating Clinical Research.* Boston: Thomson Centerwatch. 12 chapters, 7 appendices, 411 pp.

Dictionaries, Manuals, and Encyclopedias

If clinical trials are 95% tedium, then the other 5% is writing—protocols, handbooks, forms and, of course, manuscripts. No writer can expect to write with any precision without a dictionary at arm's reach. First and foremost in this collection is a standard desk dictionary. For compactness and precision, *Merriam-Webster's Collegiate Dictionary* is this writer's odds-on favorite, but many others will do. In fact, a collection of dictionaries is useful when "word shopping."

Also necessary are specialty dictionaries, books, and manuals, as listed below.

Basic Reference

Beers, Mark H.; Berkow, Robert, eds. 1999. *The Merck Manual of Diagnosis and Therapy,* 17th edition. New York: John Wiley & Sons. 2833 pp.

The Rand Corporation. 1955. *A Million Random Digits with 100,000 Normal Deviates.*New York: The Free Press (1955); Rand (2001). 628 pp.

U.S. DHHS, Office for Protection from Research Risks. *Code of Federal Regulations, Title 45: Public Welfare, Part 46:Protection of Human Subjects.* Revised 18 June 1991. Washington, DC: Office for Human Research Protections. 29 pp.

U.S. Food and Drug Administration. 2001, 2005. *Code of Federal Regulations: Title 21 Food and Drugs.* Online at http://www.access.gpo.gov/cgi-bin/cfrassemble.cgi?title=200121

http://www.accessdata.fda.gov/SCRIPs/cdrh/cfdocs/cfcfr/CRFSearch.cfm

Dictionaries

Day, Simon. 2007. *Dictionary for Clinical Trials,* 2nd edition. New York: John Wiley & Sons 249 pp.

Dorland, W.A. Newman, ed. 2000. *Dorland's Illustrated Medical Dictionary*, 29th edition. New York: WB Saunders Company. 2088 pp.

Last, John M. 2001. *A Dictionary of Epidemiology*, 4th edition. New York: Oxford University Press. 196 pp.

Last, John M. 2007. *A Dictionary of Public Health*. New York: Oxford University Press. 407 pp.

Lynch, Jack, ed. 2002. Samuel Johnson's Dictionary: Selections from the 1755 Work that Defined the English Language. DelRay Beach, FL: Levenger Press. 646 pp.

Marriott, F.H.C. 1990. *A Dictionary of Statistical Terms*, 5th edition. New York: Longman Scientific and Technical. 223 pp.

Meinert, Curtis L. 1996. *Clinical Trials Dictionary: Terminology and Usage Recommendations*. Baltimore: Harbor Duvall Graphics. 363 pp.

Mish, Frederick C., editor-in-chief. 2003. *Merriam-Webster's Collegiate Dictionary*, 11th edition. New York: Merriam-Webster, Inc. 1664 pp.

Vogt, W. Paul. 1993. *Dictionary of Statistics and Methodology*. Thousand Oaks, CA: Sage Publications. 252 pp.

Winslade, Jeffery; Hutchinson, David. 1998. *Dictionary of Clinical Research*, 2nd edition. Surrey, UK: Brookwood Medical Publications. 115 pp.

Manuals of Style

Chicago Editorial Staff. 1993. *The Chicago Manual of Style*, 14th edition. Chicago: University of Chicago Press. 921 pp.

JAMA and Archive Journals. 2007. AMA *Manual of Style: A Guide for Authors and Editors*, 10th edition. New York:Oxford University Press.1032 pp.

Strunk, William Jr.; White, E.B. 1999. *The Elements of Style*, 4th edition. New York: Longman. 105 pp.; latest edition of the original written by William Strunk Jr. and published in 1918.

Encyclopedias

Armitage, Peter; Colton, Theodore, eds. 2005. *Encyclopedia of Biostatistics*, 2nd edition. New York: John Wiley & Sons 8 vols., 6100 pp.

D'Agostino, Ralph B.; Sullivan, Lisa; Massaro, Joseph, editors-in-chief. 2008. *Wiley Encyclopedia of Clinical Trials*. New York: John Wiley & Sons. 4 vols., 2460 pp.

Codes and Guidelines

Committee on Science, Engineering, and Public Policy (P. Griffiths, chair). 1995. *On Being a Responsible Scientist*, 2nd edition. New York: National Academy Press. 40 pp.

Council for International Organizations of Medical Sciences. 2002. *International Ethical Guidelines for Biomedical Research Involving Human Subjects*. Online at www.cioms.ch. 56 pp.

Hippocrates of Cos (460–370 BC). 1910. *The Hippocratic Oath*. Classical version. Boston: Harvard Classics. Volume 39.

International Committee of Medical Journal Editors. 2004. Clinical trial registration: A statement from the International Committee of Medical Journal Editors. *JAMA* 292:1363–1364.

International Committee of Medical Journal Editors. 2007. *Uniform Requirements for Manuscripts Submitted to Biomedical Journals: Writing and Editing for Biomedical Publication*. Online at www.icmje.org. 36 pp.

Moher, David; Schultz, Kenneth F.; Altman, Douglas G., for the CONSORT Group. 2001. Revised recommendations for improving the quality of reports of parallel group randomized trials. *Lancet* 357:1191–1194.

National Commission for the Protection of Human Subjects of Biomedical and Behavioral Research (KJ Ryan, Chair). 1979. *The Belmont Report: Ethical Principles and Guidelines for the Protection of Human Subjects of Research*. Washington, DC: U.S. Government Printing Office. No. 1983-381-132:3205.

NIH Office of Extramural Research. 6 March 1998. *NIH Policy and Guidelines on the Inclusion of Children as Participants in Research Involving Human Subjects*. Online at http://grants.nih.gov/grants/guide/notice-files/not98-024.html. 8 pp.

NIH Office of Extramural Research. 10 June 1998. *NIH Policy for Data and Safety Monitoring*. Online at http://grants.nih.gov/grants/guide/notice-files/NOT98-084.html. 4 pp.

NIH Office of Extramural Research. 1994. *NIH Policy and Guidelines on the Inclusion of Women and Minorities as Subjects in Clinical Research - Amended October 2001*. Online at http://grants.nih.gov/grants/funding/women_min/guidelines_amended_10_2001.htm. 10 pp.

NIH Office of Extramural Research. 1 March 2002. *NIH Announces Draft Statement on Sharing Research Data*. Online at http://grants.nih.gov/grants/guide/notice-files/NOT-OD-02-035.html. 2 pp.

U.S. Department of Health and Human Services. 17 August 2000. Health insurance reform: Standards for electronic transactions: Announcement of designated standard maintenance organizations: Final rule and notice. *Federal Register* 65;160:50,312–50,372.

U.S. Nüremberg Military Tribunals. 1947. *The Nüremberg Code.* BMJ Vol. 313; 7 December 1996. 1 p.

World Medical Association General Assembly. 2004. *World Medical Association Declaration of Helsinki: Ethical Principles for Medical Research Involving Human Subjects.* Online at www.wma.net. 5 pp.

Examples

University Group Diabetes Program Research Group. 1970. A study of the effects of hypoglycemic agents on vascular complications in patients with adult-onset diabetes I. Design, methods, and baseline characteristics; II. Mortality results. *Diabetes* 19(Suppl 2):747–830.

Cornfield, J. 1971. The University Group Diabetes Program: A further statistical analysis of the mortality findings. *JAMA* 217:1676–1687.

Coronary Drug Project Research Group. 1973. The Coronary Drug Project: Design, methods, and baseline results. *Circulation* 47(Suppl I): I-1–I-50

Committee for the Assessment of Biometric Aspects of Controlled Trials of Hypoglycemic Agents. 1975. Report of the Committee for the Assessment of Biometric Aspects of Controlled Trials of Hypoglycemic Agents. *JAMA* 231:583–608.

Coronary Drug Project Research Group. 1983. The Coronary Drug Project: Methods and lessons of a multicenter clinical trial. *Control Clin Trials* 4: 273–549.

Hypertension Prevention Trial Research Group. 1989. The Hypertension Prevention Trial (HPT): Design, methods, and baseline results. *Control Clin Trials* 10 (Suppl)1S–117S.

Other Readings

The list below is a collection of papers and reports of historical import in the design and conduct of clinical trials.

Beecher, H.K. 1966. *Ethics and clinical research. N Engl J Med* 274:1354–1360.

Tuskegee Syphilis Study Ad Hoc Advisory Panel (Broadus N. Butler, chair). 1973.*Tuskegee Syphilis Study Ad Hoc Advisory Panel: Final Report.* Washington, DC: United States Public Health Service. 47 pp. 47

Chalmers, T.C. 1975. Randomization of the first patient. *Med Clin North Am* 59:1035–1038.

Sackett, D.L., Gent, M. 1979. Controversy in counting and attributing events in clinical trials. N Engl J Med 301:1410–1412.

Coronary Drug Project Research Group. 1980. Influence of adherence to treatment and response of cholesterol on mortality in the Coronary Drug Project. N Engl J Med 303:1038–1041.

Freedman, B. 1987. Equipoise and the ethics of clinical research. N Engl J Med 317:141–145.

Yusuf, S., Wittes, J., Probstfield, J., Tyroler, H.A. 1991. Analysis and interpretation of treatment effects in subgroups of patients in randomized clinical trials. JAMA 266:93–98.

Sobering treatise on the likelihood of subgroup differences reproduced in follow-on trials reporting subgroup differences

Committee on the Ethical and Legal Issues Relating to the Inclusion of Women in Clinical Studies (Ruth Faden and Daniel Federman, co-chairs). 1994. Women and Health Research: Ethical and Legal Issues of Including Women in Clinical Studies (in 2 volumes; 2nd volume Workshop and Commissioned Papers). New York: National Academy Press. Vol. 1., 271 pp.; vol. 2, 247 pp.

Useful discussion and recommendations relating to women in clinical trials

Meinert, C.L. 1998. Masked monitoring in clinical trials: Blind stupidity? N Engl J Med 338:1381–1382.

Institute of Medicine Committee to Review the Fialuridine (FIAU/FIAC) Clinical Trials(Morton Swartz, chair). 1995. Review of the Fialuridine (FIAU) Clinical Trials. New York: National Academy Press. 269 pp.

A series of trials that led to death and liver failure, with considerable effort devoted to faulting investigators for failure to have reported what was regarded by the U.S. Food and Drug Administration (FDA) as adverse events

A Reading List of a Different Kind

As a would-be teacher of doctoral students aspiring to be trialists, and as one often responsible for "teaching" budding researchers aiming to undertake multicenter trials, it has been useful to have a "reading list of a different kind" to aid in those efforts.

Parish, Peggy (illustrations by Fritz Siebel). 1963. Amelia Bedelia. New York: Harper Collins 64 pp.; children's book.

As it turns out, Mrs. Roberts asks Amelia to house sit while she is out running errands. Before departing she gives Amelia a list of tasks to be performed. Amelia, being a literalist, does exactly as instructed—to the consternation of Mrs. Roberts on her return. The trouble was in the instructions given, not in Amelia's execution of them. The book makes the list because it provides a sober reminder of the futility of the task of writing foolproof protocols and data collection forms immune from misinterpretation.

Merriam, Eve (retold; illustrations by Trina Schart Hyman). 1968. *Epaminondas.* New York: Follett Publishing Co. 32 pp.; children's book.

Epaminondas makes the list because the story underscores the futility of instruction when "common sense" is in short supply. Epaminondas is a little boy who applies what he is told by his mother. Problems start when his grandmother gives him a cake to carry home. By the time he gets home, he has only a handful of crumbs. His Mother is careful to explain how he should carry cake. But the next time, his grandmother gives him freshly churned butter. What he was told for carrying cake does not work well with butter! Likewise, the instruction he was given for carrying butter does not work well when it is a puppy he takes home. And the instruction for bringing a puppy home does not work when next it is a loaf of bread he has to bring home. He ties a string around it, being careful to make sure it is "not too tight and not too loose," and then drags it on home—just as his mother instructed!

Nash, Ogden (illustrations by James Marshall; 1991). 1963. *The Adventures of Isabel.* New York: Little Brown & Co. Children's book.

The Adventures of Isabel is a story of how Isabel learned to dispose of her nightmares. It makes the list because we all have nightmares to dispose of in the art and science of trials. The story was written by Ogden Nash to help his young daughter through her nightmares.*

---

* I used the story to help my own daughter deal with her nightmares. She would wake up in the middle of the night, screaming bloody murder. More often than not, before I got to her, she had her two sisters screaming in unison because, as every parent knows, screaming is contagious.

Early on, I simply comforted her and waited for her to go back to sleep, but I soon learned that she would be back to screaming an hour or so later. Eventually, I resorted to more drastic

Piper, Watty (pen name for Mabel Bragg); illustrated by Lois Lenski. 1930. *The Little Engine That Could* (aka The Pony Engine). New York: Platt & Munk; 1978 edition by Grosset & Dunlap. Children's book; 48 pp.

On the list because of the importance of the "I think I can" attitude, especially after the cars are hitched to the engine and he starts pulling them up hill—much like what happens once investigators realize how difficult it is to recruit and retain people for follow-up in trials.

Grimm, Jacob; Grimm, Wilhelm. 1812. *Hansel and Gretel (in Grimms' Fairy Tales)*.

This fairy tale story is testimony to what happens when one fails to provide an indelible trail to lead one back to the starting point and therefore a lesson in the importance of documentation.

Author unknown (probably of Russian origin). Circa 1940 in U.S. *The Little Red Hen.*

On the list because one can rewrite this children's story in the context of clinical trials, in which investigators may be hard to find to do the grunt work, but come flocking when it is time to eat the bread (i.e., have their names on publications from the trial).

---

therapy—the "circle tour." I would roust her out of bed and start walking the "circle." After each revolution in the house, I would ask "What's your name? Where are you?" and "Who am I?" We kept making the rounds until she would say with disgusted irritation "Oh Dad!" I knew then the nightmare was gone for the night and that she and I could go back to bed.

One evening, as I walked into the house from work, I heard someone reading about Isabel on TV. I called the station. To my surprise, I got in touch with the hostess of the show, a woman by the name of Nash. I told her of my interest in *Isabel* and wanted to know where I might buy a copy. The hostess said she did not know, but that I should call her brother Ogden. He would know, seeing as he wrote the story. Eventually, I worked up the courage to call the number she gave me, expecting to get a recording or answering service, but I got Ogden Nash! I told him of my own Isabel and my need for a lasting therapy.

I never forgot the lesson I learned from the contact. It was obvious that the call made his day simply by knowing that there was someone out there who appreciated his work.

Eventually, the nightmares went away, no doubt due to hundreds of readings of *Isabel*.

As an aside, I had my own encounter with Isabel. She blew into Baltimore as a tropical storm on 19 September 2003, pushing a 15-foot tidal surge in front of her. She flooded our coordinating center operations in Fells Point in Baltimore.

Robert, Henry M., III; Evans, William J.; Honemann, Daniel H.; Balch, Thomas J. 2004. *Robert's Rules of Order Newly Revised in Brief*. Cambridge, MA: Da Capo Press. 20 chapters, 200 pp.

The trialist, especially the multicenter trialist, will have spent years of his or her waking life in meetings, some seemingly endless, before the Roll Is Called up Yonder. That being so, it behooves any self-respecting trialist to be familiar with *Robert's Rules of Order,* if for no other reason than to exert control over meetings. Even if you are not a student of the rules, the likelihood, with only a modicum of studying, is that you will know more about rules than anyone else in the room and, hence, be well positioned to control the discussion (see Chapter 5).

Huff, Darrell (illustrations by Irving Geis). 1954. *How to Lie with Statistics.* New York: W. W. Norton & Co. 142 pp.

This is on the list because everybody needs to know how to lie with statistics, so as to be able pick out the liars.

Shaw, George Bernard. 1913. *The Doctor's Dilemma.*

This play focuses on the conflict of interest physicians face in, on the one hand, caring for their patients and, on the other, performing unneeded procedures to earn an income. The play makes the list because of Shaw's *Preface on Doctors.* In the 88 pages (in Penguin Books, 1954) of the preface, Shaw spares no one—not the doctors, not the epidemiologists, and not the biostatisticians.

Author unknown. *Chicken Little* (aka The Sky Is Falling, Chicken Licken, Henny Penny; from Wikipedia: Buddhist Indian folklore from the 6th century BCE).

On the list because the fable illustrates the problems that arise when jumping to conclusions based on flimsy evidence.

Aesop. *The Dog and His Shadow.*

One of many fables attributed to Aesop (purportedly a slave of African decent living in Greece; 620–560 BC), this one is about greed. The fable makes the list as a reminder to trialists not to overreach when it comes to data collection and the desire to answer too many questions.

Aesop. *The Hare and the Tortoise*.

Yet another fable attributed to Aesop, this one to illustrate that slow and steady wins the race—something worth remembering when in the middle of a trial.

Baum, L. Frank. 1900. *The Wonderful Wizard of Oz* (also the Wizard of Oz). Chicago: George M Hill Co. (original publisher; many others since)

On the list because of the magic of the Wizard in convincing the scarecrow that he had a brain—roughly akin to the task of advising graduate students, as they struggle up the ladder to completion of their dissertations.

Bayan, Rick. 1994. *Cynic's Dictionary*. New York: Hearst Books. 190 pp.

A good companion to Ambrose Bierce's *Devil's Dictionary*

Bierce, Ambrose. 1993 (reproduction of works published in 1911). *The Devil's Dictionary*. New York: Dover Publications, Inc. 145 pp.

A "modestly" cynical view of our language. On the list because, in the words of Lillian Hellman (playwright; 1905–1984), "Cynicism is an unpleasant way of saying the truth."

Truss, Lynne. 2003. *Eats, Shoots & Leaves: The Zero Tolerance Approach to Punctuation*. New York: Gotham Books. 209 pp.

Book illustrating the confusion that can arise by errant punctuation, as illustrated by the title in an errant attempt to describe the standard diet of panda bears; something to remember when writing study publications.

Carroll, Robert T. 2003. *The Skeptic's Dictionary: A Collection of Strange Beliefs, Amazing Deceptions, and Dangerous Delusions*. New York: John Wiley & Sons. 456 pp.

Butler, Ellis Parker. 1905. *Pigs is Pigs*. New York: A. L. Burt Company. 37 pp.

This children's book is on the list to illustrate the importance of definitions. The definitional problem arises when Mr. Morehouse came to the freight office to pick up a pair (a male and female) of guinea pigs for his son. Mr. Morehouse argues that the charge should be for domestic pets (25 cents each), but the railroad agent insists on charging the fare for pigs—30 cents each—and keeps the pair until the dispute can be solved.

Months later, the agent relents, but only after he had hundreds of guinea pigs in his care.

Aesop. *The Boy Who Cried Wolf* (aka *The Shepherd and the Wolf*).
    One of many fables with a moral attributed to Aesop. The fable makes the list to illustrate the consequences of fabrication.

Author unknown. *Stone Soup.*
    This children's story is about a con job done to get a meal by professing to be able to make soup from a stone. A trialist has to be able to make soup from a stone by conning for the funding needed to do the trial and then conning investigators into believing they can recruit for the trial.

Numeroff, Laura Joffe (illustrated by Felicia Bond). 1985. *If You Give a Mouse a Cookie.* New York: HarperCollins.
    On the list to illustrate that actions have consequences, hence the need to be careful in writing study protocols, lest the things proposed lead to places you do not want to go.

22

Clinical Trials and Our Health

The only way to keep your health is to eat what you don't want, drink what you don't like, and do what you'd rather not.

Mark Twain

Life expectancy at birth for people born in 2005 is estimated to be 80.4 years for females and 75.2 for males. Life expectancy is the age at which half the people born at a given point in time are expected to be still alive. Hence, at expectancies of 80.4 and 75.2 years, half of the female population is expected to live beyond 80.4 years and half the male population is expected to live beyond 75.2 years (http://www.cdc.gov/nchs/data/nvsr/nvsr56/nvsr56_10.pdf).

Life expectancy at birth in the United States (both sexes combined) was 47.3 years in 1900, 68.2 years in 1950, and 77.0 years in 2000. The increase in life expectancy in the first 50 years of the 20th century was 20.9 years and 8.8 in the second half of the 20th century. The increases correspond to an additional five months per calendar year during the first half of the 20th century and two months per calendar year in the second half (http://www.cdc.gov/nchs/data/hus/hus07.pdf#027).

The leading cause of death in 1900 was pneumonia and influenza (counted together in cause-of-death statistics). Heart disease was fourth. By 1950, pneumonia and influenza had dropped to sixth, and heart disease was first (http://www.cdc.gov/nchs/data/dvs/lead1900_98.pdf). In 2000, heart disease remained 1st and pneumonia and influenza was seventh (http://www.cdc.gov/nchs/data/dvs/LCWK9_2000.pdf).

The dramatic increase in life expectancy from 1900 to 1950 was due, in part, to attacks on infectious diseases by vaccination. The road to a vaccine against smallpox was marked by an "inoculation trial" by Lady Mary Wortley-Montague and Charles Maitland in 1721. The trial involved six inmates from the Newgate Prison. (The inmates were recruited through a policy, urged by Lady Wortley-Montague, in which King George I commuted the sentence of convicted felons if they agreed to inoculation.) Prisoners were inoculated by engrafting smallpox matter from a patient with the natural disease onto both arms and their right leg. The fact that the prisoners remained free of smallpox was taken as evidence in favor of inoculation.*[32]

Edward Jenner (1749–1823) described a series of experiments that involved a small number of people (14), who had been vaccinated with cowpox.[12] Jenner inoculated three of these people with smallpox and the others with cowpox. He subsequently wrote:

> After the many fruitless attempts to give the Small-pox to those who had had the Cow-pox, it did not appear necessary, nor was it convenient to me, to inoculate the whole of those who had been the subjects of these late trials; yet I thought it right to see the effects of variolous matter on some of them, particularly William Summers, the first of these patients who had been infected with matter taken from the cow. He was therefore inoculated with variolous matter from a fresh pustule; but, as in the preceding Cases, the system did not feel the effects of it in the smallest degree.[66]

Smallpox was officially certified by the World Health Organization (WHO) as having been eradicated in 1980.[40]

---

* The results were not as convincing as first perceived. One of the six inmates was subsequently found to have had smallpox before inoculation and a second may have had the disease in childhood.

Polio became a reportable disease in the United States in early 1900. Franklin Delano Roosevelt, the 32nd president of the United States, was afflicted with its paralyzing sequelae after he contracted the disease in 1921. (See http://www.cdc.gov/vaccines/events/polio-vacc-50th/timeline.htm for a time-line of the disease.) The disease is due to a virus, spread primarily via the fecal–oral route. Infections with the virus are largely asymptomatic, especially if encountered early in life. The exposure to the wild virus diminished with the advent of indoor plumbing. As a consequence, "natural immunization" diminished, and the population of susceptibles increased, thus leading to epidemics of the disease by the 1940s. At the height of the epidemic in 1952, there were 57,879 cases of polio reported and 3,145 deaths attributed to the disease (http://www.cdc.gov/vaccines/pubs/pinkbook/downloads/appendices/G/cases&deaths.pdf).

Although a relatively minor disease in terms of mortality, it was a major disease in the emotional burden it exacted because of its propensity to strike children. Parents prohibited their children from the usual joys of summer like swimming, picnics, movies, and community gatherings. Every child was schooled as to the presenting symptoms of the disease and to report them to their parents in the hope that early diagnosis would spare the child the paralyzing sequelae of the disease. Indeed, there were any number of summer mornings in the early 1950s when I awoke with a stiff neck sufficient to convince me that I contracted the dreaded disease.

Eventually, the work of Jonas Salk and others led to a killed-virus vaccine, culminating in a massive nationwide field trial in 1954. Results of the trial were reported April 12, 1955, at the University of Michigan, with the conclusion that the vaccine was safe and effective.[70] The vaccine was approved for general use within days after the announcement, and mass immunization commenced that year.* In 1988, the WHO set a goal for the

---

* The 1954 field trial involved 1.8 million children in 44 states. Children in the first, second, and third grades in 13 states willing to be randomized were assigned to receive the vaccine or a matching placebo. Children in the second grade in schools in the other 33 states received the vaccine, and children in the first and third grades in participating schools served as observed controls. There were about 600,000 children in the randomized trial and about 1.2 million children in the nonrandomized component of the field trial.

worldwide eradication of polio. The disease has not yet been eradicated, but is well on its way to extinction.

The human immunodeficiency virus (HIV) has replaced polio on the emotional worry list. The virus was first identified by a French scientist in 1983 and is now pandemic. Infection occurs from transfer of bodily fluids from persons infected with the virus to uninfected people. HIV infection, in the early days of the burgeoning epidemic, was akin to a death sentence, to the extent that infection led to acquired immune deficiency syndrome (AIDS), a set of symptoms resulting from damage to the immune system caused by HIV, and death. But, thanks to massive research efforts, leading eventually to highly active antiretroviral therapy (HAART), HIV infection today is akin to living with a chronic disease. Life expectancy for people with AIDS has increased from less than a year to several years, thanks to HAART and various other treatments.

Some advances are so gradual that they go largely unnoticed, until one looks. Childhood cancers are dreadful. Parents never recover from the death of a child, whatever the cause. (I know because my mother would tear up in her 80s every time Maynard's name came up—a brother I never knew who died of a brain tumor before I was born.)

The incidence of childhood cancers has increased from 1975 to 1995, but mortality rates have declined. The age-adjusted mortality rate (all races, both sexes, age <20) fell from 50 deaths/million population to 30 deaths in the interval (in contrast to a 20-point increase in incidence; 130 cases per million population to 150 cases in the 20-year period).[110]

Female mortality from invasive breast cancer has declined from 1975 to 2005. Age-adjusted rates per 100,000 population fell from 31.4 to 24.0 (http://seer.cancer.gov/csr/1975_2005/results_merged/sect_04_breast.pdf; Table IV-4). The decline is due to improved screening and diagnostic procedures, improved treatment procedures, and improved postdiagnostic care and treatment emanating, in large measure, from the National Surgical Adjuvant and Bowel Project (NSABP)—one of the cooperative groups funded by the National Cancer Institute (http://www.nsabp.pitt.edu/NSABP_Protocols.asp).

Mortality rates from heart disease in the United States in 2005 are about one-third of what they were in 1950, as seen in the table below (data from http://www.cdc.gov/nchs/data/hus/hus07.pdf).

Age-adjusted mortality rates for heart disease; U.S. population; 1950 and 2005; rates per 100,000 population

	1950	2005	Difference	% drop
Both sexes	586.8	211.1	375.7	64.0
Male	697.0	260.9	436.1	62.6
Female	484.7	172.3	312.4	61.5

The decline is due, no doubt, to a host of reasons, but certainly randomized treatment and prevention trials have a prominent place in the list of credits for the reduction. The percentage drop in mortality has been the same for both sexes (last column in the table). This reality should give pause to those who have argued that women have been deprived of the benefits of heart trials because they involved mostly males.

Clearly, we benefit from information generated from trials, whether or not we participate in them. This argues for a mind-set akin to that regarding jury duty. Most of us hope that we will not be called, but we also recognize that we have a duty to serve if called. By analogy, if we want our system of research to work, we have to do our fair share to make sure that it does. That means, when it comes to participation in trials for which we are eligible, we should be willing to consider such participation. The efficiency of trials and the speed at which information is generated is a direct function of the time and energy it takes to enroll participants. The sooner they are enrolled, the better it is for all of us.

23

Final Exam

You cannot learn anything with your mouth open.

CLM

Now there is just one thing remaining: A final exam. The mere mention of the words still sends chills down my spine! Below is a set of 50 true-or-false questions and ten multiple-choice questions. Go through, answer them (without looking at the answers), and see how you do.

If you manage to answer every question wrong, you are on the right track. You just have to invert your thinking. If you got half right using the Charlie Brown method of answering, you did about as well as you can expect. If you got every one right, you are good to go! If you still have the energy, finish off by testing your wits on *Clinical Trials Trivia*.

True\False Quiz

1. Randomization is done to ensure comparable treatment groups. . . . .(T) (F)

False (see Chapter 11). If you want comparability, you have to help randomization along with stratification, but the trouble is that you can only stratify on one or two variables. Stratify on too many variables and it is like not stratifying at all. Besides, stratification does nothing to improve the precision of treatment comparisons if the variables used for stratification do not influence the outcome of interest (usually the way it turns out).

In many senses, stratification as a means of variance control is overrated. If a trial involves only a dozen people or so, stratification for variance control will be ineffective. If it involves 100 or more people, it is unnecessary.

2. Stratification on gender is done to ensure that the treatment groups have the same number of females as males.... (T) (F)

False. It is done to make sure the treatment groups have the same proportionate mix of males to females. Stratification has nothing to do with ensuring equal numbers.

3. If only a small number of females is expected in a trial, they should be excluded because there will not be enough females for meaningful analyses.......................... (T) (F)

False. Not unless there are medical-legal reasons to do so. There is a difference between *designed subgroup comparisons* and *ad hoc subgroup comparisons*. A designed subgroup comparison involves set sample size requirements for the subgroups to be compared when the trial is designed. Ad hoc subgroup comparisons involve whatever sample sizes are achieved when recruitment is finished.

The difference is that, in the former comparison, the power for a gender-by-treatment comparison is specified at design time, whereas in the latter approach, it is whatever it is at analysis time.

The most efficient strategy is a "floating" enrollment economy. In regard to gender, that means taking whoever is eligible and letting the gender mix be what it is.

One of the cause célèbre "male-only" trials serving to reinforce the view that women were excluded from trials was the Physicians Health Study (PHS)—a primary prevention trial of male physicians aged 40 to 84. The trial served to help establish the value of a baby aspirin a day as a preventative for myocardial infarction (MI). The PHS was designed to involve both male and female physicians, but was ultimately limited to males because of concern of the study section reviewing the application that the number of female physicians[105] (about one in ten when the trial was done) was not large enough to provide reliable information on possible treatment differences by gender.

4. The Tuskegee Syphilis Study was a trial involving poor black males. . . . . (T) (F)

False. A trick question! The Tuskegee Syphilis Study was, indeed, a study involving poor black males, but it was not a trial. It was a follow-up study. All trials are part of the class of follow-up studies (they all involve cohorts of people and follow-up), but not all cohort follow-up studies are trials.

The study started in 1932; it was located in Macon County, Alabama; was endorsed by the Tuskegee Institute (a historically black institute); and was funded by the U.S. Public Health Service (USPHS). It was motivated by observations that syphilis in blacks appeared to be more virulent than in whites, a situation not unlike today's arguments that heart disease in women is different from that seen in men. The outcry regarding the study was triggered by a story in the *New York Times* (July 26, 1972) revealing that people in the study were not offered treatment—penicillin—when it became available after World War II.

The outrage from the revelation helped derail the nomination of Henry Foster for U.S. Surgeon General in 1995, when it was revealed that he had known about the study several years before his nomination and had not voiced objections to it. (More importantly, Foster's nomination was overturned by the fact he, an ob-gyn physician, had performed a number of "pregnancy terminations," ranging in number, depending on source, from a high of 700 to a low of 39.)

President Clinton issued an apology for the study on behalf of the nation in 1997.

5. Only subgroups specified when a trial is designed should be examined for treatment differences. . . . . (T) (F)

False! The trialist is obliged to look for subgroup differences before reporting results, if only to be satisfied that no notable subgroup differences exist (i.e., to be satisfied that the treatment effect being reported is homogeneous across subgroups represented in the trial).

Do not confuse subgroup analyses, done to ensure that the conclusion regarding the main effect is reasonable with *data dredging*, done to find "significant" differences (see Chapters 11 and 17).

6. Randomization is necessary for ensuring the validity of trials. . . . . (T) (F)

False. A trial is valid if the most parsimonious explanation of the results (i.e., the explanation requiring the fewest assumptions) is treatment assignment (the experimental variable). The purpose of randomization is to remove selection bias from the assignment process. Absent randomization, it is difficult to rule out selection bias as the explanation of the results observed.

One should not assume that randomized trials are valid and that all other are invalid. The proof is in the pudding.

7. Trials have to have representative study populations to be generalizable. . . . . (T) (F)

False. Generalizations are matters of judgment, except when it is possible to select people for study at random—not possible in any study for which consents are required—and hence always done at the risk of being wrong. They are made less risky with randomization because the generalization is to the treatment effect, to the biology of the treatment effect, if you will. Hence, a treatment that exerts an effect can be reasonably expected to have that effect in all people sharing a common biology. So, for example, to the extent that males and females are alike biologically, one can generalize across genders, even if only males or only females are studied. We often generalize from adults to children when it comes to use of drugs in children, when most of the testing was done on adults.

8. Phase IV drug trials are done after a drug has been approved for marketing. . . . . (T) (F)

True (see Chapter 1 for definition). Phase IV trials (not to be confused with postmarketing surveillance studies) are typically done under circumstances approximating real-world conditions; usually with a clinical event as the outcome of interest, designed for long-term treatment (when appropriate) and follow-up; and to assess efficacy and safety of the drug against a designated control treatment.

9. Most phase IV trials are done by drug companies. . . . . (T) (F)

False. Once a drug has been approved, companies have little incentive to do such trials. For example, the University Group Diabetes Program (UGDP), as discussed in Chapter 15, was sponsored by the National Institutes of Health (NIH) because there was nothing to be gained by companies marketing antidiabetic drugs in supporting such a trial, seeing as such drugs were already licensed for use in blood sugar control.

10. Most drug trials are funded by the U.S. Food and Drug Administration (FDA). . . . . (T) (F)

False. The FDA has only a modest research budget.

11. Results during a trial should not be analyzed because doing so will screw-up p-values. . . . . (T) (F)

False. If doing so screws up p-values, too bad for p-values. Preserving p-value pales in importance when measured against the need to make certain people are not being harmed during the trial.

12. Monitoring for treatment differences during a trial should be done using preordained stopping rules. . . . . (T) (F)

The answer depends on who you ask. False if you ask me. To be sure, there are trials in which monitoring is done with stopping rules, but in most cases the rules are more like guidelines than rules. With a rule, stop is automatic when the conditions of the rule are met. Halting the study is not automatic with the use of stopping guidelines.

Stopping rules are mostly p-value–based for a test statistic evaluated at predetermined points during the course of the trial.[99] A difference exceeding a set limit leads to termination of one of the study treatments, depending on the nature and direction of the observed treatment difference.

13. The purpose of randomization is to remove selection bias from the treatment assignment process. . . . . (T) (F)

True. It has other benefits, but that is its primary benefit.

14. The first randomized trials were done in the 1960s.........(T) (F)
False. Much earlier, in the 1920s and '30s.

15. Most clinical trials are positive........................(T) (F)
False. Don't we wish the answer to be true? The likelihood is that, if we were able to know the result of every trial undertaken, whether published or not, most are nil simply because most trials are too small to detect differences, even if they exist. Even in published trials, a fair number are nil or negative.* For example, of the 80 multicenter randomized trials published in the *New England Journal of Medicine* in 2006, 27 were classified as negative or nil.

16. The state of clinical equipoise is necessary
for the conduct of trials. ....(T) (F)
False. Equipoise is necessary for the ethical conduct of superiority trials but does not exist for trials done to show equivalence or noninferiority (see Chapter 8 for discussion of clinical equipoise and Chapter 7 for types of trials).

17. Treatment effects monitoring (aka data and safety monitoring)
should be done in masked fashion........................(T) (F)
The answer depends on who you ask, but if you ask me my answer is "false" for reasons enunciated in reference 82.

Masking monitors means that they are in the dark as to whether an emerging treatment difference is positive or negative (i.e., whether it is indicative of benefit or harm). Masked monitoring is predicated on the assumption that the sign of a treatment difference is irrelevant in deciding whether or not to recommend a protocol change in the trial. That is to say, the same size treatment difference, whether positive or negative, will lead to a recommendation of a protocol change. However, as a rule, differences against the test treatment will lead to protocol changes sooner than will

---

* "Negative," in relation to results from a trial, can mean the absence of an effect or the presence of one opposite to the one expected or desired. "Negative" and "nil" are used here to differentiate between the two effects.

differences in favor of the test treatment. Why? Because, bad effects are immediate, whereas there is the possibility that positive effects can be offset later on by ill effects; hence, a tendency to wait longer before acting to make certain the effect is real. If you want to read more on masking monitors see reference 82.

18. Most trials are done on males. . . . . (T) (F)
    False: see Chapter 7.

19. Most clinical trials are undertaken in the hope of showing benefits. . . . . (T) (F)
    True (but, most assuredly, they don't always turn out that way). Of the 111 randomized trials published in the *New England Journal of Medicine* in 2006, all but three were classified as superiority trials.

20. "Intention to treat" (ITT) is jargon for "analysis by treatment assignment." . . . . (T) (F)
    True.

21. If treatment effects monitoring is done, the number of looks allowed should be specified before "looking" starts. . . . . (T) (F)
    False, if you ask me, for the same reason stated in the answer to Question 17. That approach does not pass the Mother Test (see Appendix A).
    Suppose you see an emerging trend and there is need to look again, sooner than planned. Are you going to prohibit that because another look cannot occur until months hence? Not wise.

22. A person who refuses the treatment assignment should be dropped from analysis. . . . . (T) (F)
    False. Not if analyses are by "intention to treat."

23. The usual approach to recruitment is to enroll equal numbers of males and females. . . . . (T) (F)
    False. The usual approach is to enroll without regard to gender (or any other subgroup, for that matter). The obvious difficulty with enrollment

quotas is that it takes longer to complete enrollment (to say nothing of the ethical implications in excluding persons on the basis of some characteristic because the quota has been reached with regard to, say, gender) if the male–female mix of study-eligible people is markedly different (often the case).

**24. "New drug" and "new compound" are synonymous
in the parlance of the FDA..** . . . . (T) (F)
False. See discussion in Chapter 3.

25. Treatment-by-gender interactions are rare in trials. . . . . (T) (F)
True. By and large, even if interactions exist, they are hellishly difficult to detect. The reality is that most trials are not large enough to detect main effects, let alone interaction effects.

The inability to detect interactions does not mean they do not exist. It simply means they are not detectable within the limits of the trial. That said, it must also be recognized that the biological characteristics contributing to gender-by-treatment interactions are not as common as people preoccupied with gender differences would have you believe.

**26. Changing dates recorded for clinic visits so forms
can be keyed is OK.** . . . . (T) (F)
Please tell me you checked false! Any such change constitutes falsification and is research misconduct—conduct that has serious consequences, including potential for dismissal and debarment.

Information keyed must correspond to data in the patient's medical record. The temptation to make such changes comes from time windows around visits and data entry systems in which a visit is counted as missed if not done within the time window. See Chapters 8 and 11 (Myth 16) for more.

**27. Journal editors are the major contributors to publication
bias because of their tendency to reject "negative" studies..** . . . . . (T) (F)
False. The largest contributors to the bias are researchers who fail to write up negative or nil studies for publication.

28. Membership on institutional review boards (IRBs) is
limited to people from the institutions they represent. . . . . (T) (F)
    False. By law, IRBs must be comprised of at least one person without
any institutional affiliation.[100]

29. A clinical trial is an experiment involving human beings. . . . (T) (F)
    True. The term applies even if the trial is in-vitro, so long as it involves
tissue from human beings. Technically, the term applies to studies done in
animals as well. For example, PubMed, as of August 6, 2008, has 18,697
publications indexed to "clinical trial" tagged "animal" (compared to 528,971
tagged "human").

30. The Nüremberg Code was an outgrowth of the first meeting
of the World Medical Council in Nüremberg, in 1963. . . . . (T) (F)
    False. It was an outgrowth of the Nüremberg War Crimes Trials after
World War II.

31. External validity and generalizability mean
the same thing.. . . . . (T) (F)
    True. The epidemiologist speaks of external validity, and the trialist
speaks of generalizability, but they mean the same thing.

32. Institutional review board approvals are good for
the life of a project. . . . . (T) (F)
    False. They have to be renewed; typically annually, but the review and
approval cycle may be for shorter periods of time at the discretion of the
IRB if the research is considered risky.

33. Subgroup analyses are necessary in trials. . . . . (T) (F)
    True. See Chapter 17 and Question 5.

34. "Data dredging" is a pejorative for "subgroup analysis.". . . . (T) (F)
    False. See Chapter 17 and Question 5.

35. Trialists should stratify randomizations if a qualitative interaction is expected. . . . . (T) (F)

False. A qualitative interaction is one in which the treatment is beneficial in one group and harmful in the complement of that group (e.g., males vs. females). If that is the case, the proper design strategy is to exclude the subgroup in which the treatment is assumed to be harmful, for obvious medical and ethical reasons.

36. James Lind is famous for having done the first trial for treatment of rickets. . . . . (T) (F)

False. His trial had to do with scurvy. See Chapter 1.

37. The most common punishment for fraud in research is fine and imprisonment. . . . . (T) (F)

False. The most common punishment is debarment for a period of time, in which persons found guilty of scientific misconduct are barred from research.

38. The Belmont Report is a report on the state of clinical trials, published in 1979. . . . . (T) (F)

False. It was published in 1979 alright, but it is about the ethics of performing research upon human beings (see Chapter 8).

39. By tradition, the baseline period of observation ends on the seventh day following randomization. . . . . (T) (F)

False. The baseline period of observation for a person ends when treatment assignment is issued for the person.

40. A person should be counted as enrolled when the treatment assignment is revealed to clinic personnel. . . . . . . (T) (F)

True! Keep in mind that "revealed" does not mean that clinic personnel know the treatment being administered; the treatment is not known if assignments are masked, as in double-masked trials.

41. Randomization is done to protect against
treatment-related selection bias. . . . . (T) (F)
True! Broadly, bias related to treatment assignment occurs when investigators know treatment assignments in advance of issue and use that information in deciding who to select and when to enroll them.

42. Patients who drop out should be replaced. . . . . (T) (F)
False. Doing so may be aesthetically pleasing, but there is no "replacing" someone who drops out. They all count. The practice is deceptive, to the extent that it encourages researchers to concentrate on "completers" while sweeping "noncompleters" under the rug.

43. The majority of trials done involve crossover designs. . . . . . . (T) (F)
False, but information supporting the answer is hard to come by. There is no way to ascertain treatment structures with indexing done by the National Library of Medicine (NLM), and who knows about trials done but never published? The predominant design is one involving parallel (uncrossed) treatment groups (see Chapter 1). Hints at an answer can be gleaned from trials registered at www.clinicaltrials.gov. The search term "cross-over" or "crossover" yields 7,071 hits vs. 39,479 for "parallel" (as of October 14, 2010).

44. The majority of clinical trials are randomized. . . . . (T) (F)
Don't we wish. Judging from counts in PubMed, less than half (248,941/528,971) are indexed to the publication type "randomized controlled trial" out of the larger publication type "clinical trial" (as of August 6, 2008).

45. A "clinical trial," by definition, involves at least
two treatment groups. . . . . (T) (F)
False. Not by the general definition used by the NLM for indexing (see Chapter 1); there, the definition includes trials involving just one group. However, randomized controlled trials will involve two or more treatment groups.

46. The purpose of treatment effects monitoring is to
protect patients from harm............................. (T) (F)
   True.

47. Research that is classified as "exempt" does not
have to be reviewed by IRBs............................ (T) (F)
   False. The classification is made by IRBs and, hence, has to be reviewed by IRBs in order to make the determination. The classification means investigators do not have to submit applications for renewal of approvals once a project is classified as "exempt." See Question 32.

48. Blocking and stratification serve the same purpose......... (T) (F)
   False. Stratification in trials is done to ensure balance in the mix of people across treatment groups (see Question 2). Blocking is done to ensure the assignment ratio is satisfied at intervals over the period of recruitment (see Chapter 2).

49. Events occurring after randomization, but before
treatment has been initiated should be ignored. .... (T) (F)
   False. Analysis should be by original treatment assignment and should include all events, regardless of when they occur after randomization.

50. Too many pigs under the same blanket and
they all get away. .... (T) (F)
   True, always! One pig per blanket!

Multiple Choice

1. Principles set forth in the Belmont Report include: (check all that apply)

   ( ) Principle of beneficence
   ( ) Principle of justice
   ( ) Principle of respect for persons

( ) Principle of medical competencies
( ) Principle of clinical equipoise

The first three.

2. The Helsinki Code is a code about: (check one)

( ) Medical ethics
( ) Good laboratory procedures
( ) Harmonization requirement for global drug testing
( ) None of the above

Medical ethics.

3. Which of the following passes for randomization? (check all that apply)

( ) Coin flips
( ) Table of random numbers
( ) Odd–even (e.g., persons seen on odd-numbered days assigned to the test treatment; persons seen on even numbered-days assigned to the control treatment)
( ) Sequential assignment (e.g., every other person seen assigned to the test treatment)
( ) None of the above
( ) All of the above

Coin flips and table of random numbers.

4. "Concealment" in regard to randomization refers to: (check one)

( ) Masked treatment administration
( ) Keeping assignments secret until issued
( ) Obscuring the lot number on study medications
( ) Masked data monitoring

Keeping assignments secret until issued, so that no one can know what is coming next; not to be confused with masked treatment administration (see Question 40).

5. A placebo patient is: (check one)

( ) One who is receiving the placebo treatment
( ) One who is no longer receiving the study treatment
( ) One who refuses the assigned treatment
( ) A hypothetical person
( ) None of the above

I hope you checked "a hypothetical person." There are "placebo-assigned patients" but no "placebo patients" in trials (unless they have been sugar-coated).

6. Ways to avoid selection bias in trials include: (check all that apply)

( ) Randomization
( ) Stratification
( ) Screening logs
( ) All of the above
( ) None of the above

Randomization.

7. Of the following, which, if any, can be done without IRB approval? (check one)

( ) Approaching persons for study
( ) Collecting data to assess eligibility for study
( ) Addition of a new examination procedure
( ) Stopping a treatment regimen because of harmful effects
( ) None of the above

Stopping a treatment regimen because of harmful effects. Harm is harm. It does not make sense to continue a bad treatment until an IRB acts. The delay, even if only a few days (likely more), serves to expose people to more risk of harm.

8. "Intention to treat" is jargon for: (check one)

( ) Analysis by original treatment assignment
( ) Analysis excluding people not eligible for study
( ) Analysis per protocol
( ) None of the above

The first item.

9. A parallel treatment design is one in which: (check one)

( ) Persons are enrolled and followed as pairs
( ) Two similar trials done at the same time
( ) People receive the same treatments but in different orders
( ) Persons receive only one of the study treatments

You are correct if you checked the last item.

10. A sequential trial is one in which: (check one)

( ) Treatments are tested in sequence
( ) Patients receive treatment in a specified sequence
( ) Sample size is not fixed
( ) Doses are escalated over time

The third item. Sample size in sequential trials is a function of the results observed and hence not fixed.

Clinical Trials Trivia

1. **Why are British sailors called limeys?** Because of James Lind and the finding that eating fresh fruits such as oranges, lemons, and limes prevented scurvy in sailors at sea (see Chapter 1).
2. **What do Henry Kissinger and the UGDP have in common?** The court cases for Henry Kissinger's telephone logs while Secretary of

State and for raw data from the UGDP coalesced to be heard together by the U.S. Supreme Court in the fall of 1979; it was decided March 1980 (6 to 2 decision against the requests), forever linking the UGDP and Henry Kissinger.[121]

3. **Who was James Lind?** A British naval surgeon (1716–1794).

4. **Where did Lind do his "scurvy trial"?** On board the HMS *Salisbury* at sea, in 1747; the *Salisbury* was a 50-foot gunship launched 1746.

5. **What is the National Commission for the Protection of Human Subjects of Biomedical and Behavioral Research known for?** For production of *The Belmont Report: Ethical Principles and Guidelines for the Protection of Human Subjects of Research* (1979); it sets forth the principles of beneficence, justice, and respect for persons in relation to research upon human beings.[93]

6. **Why is it called the "Belmont Report"?** Because the Commission produced the report while working at the Belmont Conference Center in Elkridge, Maryland.

7. **What does ITT stand for?** Intention to treat (see Chapter 2).

8. **When did the British Navy stock its ships at sea with fresh citrus fruits?** About 50 years after Lind's experiment. So much for the impact of trials on practice. The primary reason had to do with cost. Today, we think that limes grow in supermarkets, but supplying ships at sea with fresh fruit was complicated and expensive back then.

9. **What does OHRP stand for?** Office for Health Research Protections.

10. **What does it do?** Regulates IRBs.

11. **What is the largest trial ever done?** The Salk polio vaccine trial done in 1954 and 1955.

12. **How many people did it involve?** Almost 2 million people.

24

Last Words

Too many pigs under the same blanket and they all get away.

CLM

"Clinical trial" (human, English-language), as a publication type in the National Library of Medicine (NLM)'s indexing of publications in PubMed, represented 2.1% of 1966 publications and 7.7% of 2006 publications. The publication type "randomized controlled trial" was 12.3% of the publication type "clinical trial" in 1966 and 47.4% of that publication type in 2006.

The randomized trial reigns supreme for comparative evaluations. It is regarded as the gold standard for comparison of treatments, and is the lynchpin for evidence-based medicine. That being so, it is appropriate to finish this treatise with a few topics and issues related to the randomized trial, including things needing to be "fixed" and observations on some worrisome trends.

The Limits of Randomized Trials

Only a narrow set of questions can be addressed via randomized trials. For example, it would be great to know whether exposure of children to violence on TV increases their tendency to violence as adults, but such trials would be impossible—first and foremost because the notion of randomizing children to TV venues is reprehensible, to say nothing about impractical. And second because, even if there were a way around the ethical questions concerning randomization, the trials would have to be large and run for the course of a lifetime, making them prohibitively expensive.

The other reality, sticking to questions that can be addressed by randomization, is that the window of opportunity for randomizing is narrow, slamming shut sometimes before any trials are done. It closes as soon as a treatment is regarded as standard of care, even if the evidence for such a standard is lacking. A legitimate state of doubt (clinical equipoise) must exist to justify randomizing people to treatment. If there is no doubt, there is no ethical base for randomization.

Once the window closes, all that can be done is to wait. The window may reopen years later, long after a treatment first appears on the scene. The natural history of a fair number of treatments is early acceptance, followed by widespread use. Then, years later, doubts as to its merits emerge. Then, after a rising tide of doubts, the randomized trials begin. Finally, results that are nil or negative come in, and a slow decline of the treatment to oblivion occurs.

Trials and Adverse Effects

A reality about trials is that they are weak instruments for finding adverse effects. Drugs approved by the U.S. Food and Drug Administration (FDA) as "safe and effective" are only safe within the limits of detection in trials. Even in trials that involve extended periods of treatment and follow-up, there is virtually no chance of detecting rare events.

Trials, no matter how large they may become or how long they may run in the future, will remain weak in this regard. This means that we have to live with the risks of bad effects coming to light years after drugs come into use. There will be disasters, such as those that occurred with fen-phen and diethylstilbestrol (DES) in the future. Only the names will change.

Fen-phen—fenfluramine and phentermine—is a combination drug used for appetite suppression. Phentermine was approved for short-term appetite suppression in 1959; fenfluramine was approved in 1973 (http://www.fda.gov/Cder/news/phen/fenphenqa2.htm). Years later (July 1997), after widespread usage, physicians at the Mayo Clinic reported 24 cases of heart valve disease in people on fen-phen for weight control.[25] The finding led to the voluntary withdrawal of the drugs from the market in September 1997, but only after millions of prescriptions had been written.

The DES story is even more disconcerting because the adverse effect from use appeared a generation later, when female offspring of mothers treated with the synthetic estrogen reached reproductive age. Diethylstilbestrol came into use in the late 1940s as a presumed preventative against spontaneous abortion. Its use came to an end following a report of a case-control study by Herbst and Scully[58] (1970), in which they implicated use of DES in mothers of seven young women having vaginal clear-cell adenocarcinomas—a cancer rarely seen in young women. The drug was withdrawn from the market in 1971. (See reference 64 for an excellent account of the DES story.)

The fen-phen disaster emerged after widespread off-label use of these drugs, which were approved for short-term use, but were used long term and in combinations not tested in any trials.

The DES story is the result of widespread use without evidence that the drug was useful in preventing spontaneous abortion. A small trial involving 93 pregnant women published in 1952 failed to produce "evidence that diethylstilbestrol increased the pregnancy salvage rate."[112]

Authors of a much larger randomized placebo-controlled trial involving a total of 1,646 pregnant women reported the same thing the following year. They concluded that, "Stilbestrol did not reduce the incidence of abortion, prematurity, or postmaturity."[36] Obviously, neither trial was sufficient to dissuade ob-gyn physicians from using the drug in women threatening abortion.

Trials and Institutional Review Boards

The *institutional* in institutional review board means that IRBs exist within institutions and that investigators in those institutions are accountable to those IRBs, and those alone. Every IRB is autonomous and beholden to no other IRB.

The system is ill-suited for dealing with multicenter research. In regard to multicenter trials, the structure means that there can be as many IRBs to clear as there are centers in trials. Investigators at institutions not having an IRB may be directed to a commercial IRB, serving, in effect, as a central IRB, but investigators at institutions with IRBs do not have that option. The requirement of multiple independent reviews adds to the time and cost required for implementation of trials.

The IRB system came into being in the 1970s, when the majority of research was still single-centered. The world of research has become much more multicentered since then. The IRB structures need to be updated to reflect that reality.

Trials As an Academic Enterprise

There is no academic home for trialists. They are scattered throughout departments of schools of medicine and schools of public health, without a critical mass anywhere, and usually without much interaction. The scattering and lack of interaction is hindering the development of the field of clinical trials into a bona fide scientific discipline. There is no doubt that the establishment of departments of biostatistics and epidemiology in the last century helped promote those activities to science status. One can hope that there will be similar developments for trialists sometime in this century.

The Training of Trialists

The infrastructure need for doing trials depends on a cadre of people trained in the art and science of trials. That training requires a "laboratory," something akin to the way in which laboratory scientists are trained, except that in trials the "laboratory" is the coordinating center. Sustaining such activities in academic settings requires institutions with the will, resources, and wherewithal to maintain such operations. That is becoming increasingly more difficult, with the movement of many of the functions of coordinating centers to contract research organizations (CROs). Typically, the indirect costs for CROs are lower than for academic institutions.

Investigator-initiated Trials

A disquieting trend, as trials have gotten larger and more expensive, is the diminishing role of investigators in the initiation of trials. Most of the large-scale, long-term, National Institutes of Health (NIH)-funded trials initiated in the 1960s and 1970s came about as a result of investigator initiatives via the grant application process.

That mode of initiation has gotten more difficult. Starting in 1993, investigators wanting to submit grant applications with budgets of $500,000 or more in direct costs in any year of requested support must obtain permission to submit such applications. Without permission, applications will likely be returned unreviewed (per *Guidance for Principal Investigators on the Preparation of Investigator-Initiated Research Grant Applications Requesting More Than $500,000 in Direct Costs in Any Year*; NIH Guide; vol. 22, December 17, 1993).

As a result (and the usual difficulties of getting fundable priority scores for "big-ticket" items), investigators are increasingly content to rely on sponsors for initiating large-scale trials. The downside of that tendency is where it leads—to a future in which sponsors set the research agenda. The nation needs a spirited, strong-willed investigatorship to fight for research not favored by government or industry sponsors.

The Separation of Investigators from Their Results

The practice in randomized trials, especially in large-scale multicenter trials, is to shield study investigators from interim results. This shielding means that investigators do not see results by treatment group until the trial is finished.

Shielding has come about as a result of concerns that knowledge of interim results by those doing the trial may bias the results of the trial.

It is imposed to bolster the trappings of objectivity, but at the expense of the science of trials and at potential risk to those people being studied.

The fact that shielding is at odds with the usual practice in research—in which those doing the research see results as they emerge—sets trials apart from other areas of research. The fact that investigators in trials cannot be trusted to see their own data, for fear that being able to do so will bias the results, tends to cause other researchers to view clinical trials as not "real" research. That works to investigators' disadvantage, especially when standing before promotions committees.

Shielding leaves trials open to questions on medical-legal grounds because it requires investigators to assign an inalienable duty—namely, to protect those they study from harm—to others; in multicenter trials, typically, this is a monitoring body comprised of members not associated with the trial and not accountable to any IRB. That inalienable duty is implied in the Nüremberg Code and all ethical codes since Nüremberg. It is an explicit requirement of IRBs. Investigators are first in line for censure or retribution if things go wrong in the research they head.

It is a given that those who develop the protocol and collect the data are in the best position to understand and interpret the data they generate. Denying them access to interim results by treatment group reduces their ability to identify and deal with issues signaled by data and their ability to spot signals suggestive of harm to those being studied.

Objectivity should not be imposed at the expense of competency. A reasonable balance of the two requirements in multicenter trials is to compose monitoring committees of two kinds of members. Voting members, independent of the trial, and a matching number of nonvoting members from the study, in which the entire membership, voting and nonvoting, is privy to all discussions and deliberations (i.e., absent executive sessions, in which nonvoting members are excluded).

Masked Monitoring?

A practice, increasingly common in trials with monitoring committees, is to mask them to treatment group, so that the interim looks are without knowledge of treatment group. The masking is achieved by preparing reports that show results by treatment group using arbitrary labels, like A and B, to identify those groups. The purpose is to increase objectivity by forcing members to look at differences without knowing whether they are for or against the study treatment.

Carried to its extreme, this process has the potential of satisfying the jocular definition of a triple-masked trial: One where no one knows what is going on; not the patient, not the study physician, and not the statistician. The work-around to avoid that situation is to lift the mask if differences emerge in which it is important to know treatment. But, with that being the usual modus operandi, "Why mask at all"? If there are no differences, there is little to be objective about, and when there are differences, and perhaps worries about objectivity, the mask is lifted.

The masking is open to question because it reduces the individual and collective competency of the monitoring committee process.[82] The masking is implemented in the mistaken belief that "it can't hurt, so why not?" But there are costs overlooked in the push for objectivity. Masking makes it more difficult to prepare monitoring reports, it increases the risk of error in the display of data, and it limits the exploration of study data. From these perspectives, this masking is perhaps best left undone. It might well be, were it not for sponsors who believe it to be a good idea.

Final Words for Readers

For aspiring students: Pay attention.
For trialists: May all your trials be good and your tribulations few.

Appendix A

The Mother Test for Designers of Trials

Sure, fathers are great, but mothers are special.

How many times have you seen 300-pound tackles mouth "Hi, Dad!" in front of the TV camera on football fields? How many residents in nursing home call out for Dad? Who do you call when you need a shoulder to cry on? Who do you call when you just want to talk? Mom, of course!

Because mothers are our most prized possession, in trials, they provide an internal compass for gauging the adequacy of the planned trial and its conduct.

Technically, the Mother Test comes down to a single question: "Would you enroll your mother in the trial?" If your answer is *no*, you need to work to change the design and conduct procedures so you can answer *yes*, or you need to walk away from the trial.

The expectation is that, as a designer, you will be able to answer all the questions below in the affirmative. Questions answered "no" serve to identify areas in need of change or "fixing."

The essence of the Mother Test is contained in question 40 below: "Assuming your mother is eligible and willing to be enrolled into the trial, would you be willing to randomize her to treatment and to have her treated and followed as proposed?" If, as a designer or conductor of that trial, the answer is "no," you should indicate your reasons and work to change the design and conduct procedures so as to be able to answer "yes" to the question. The goal should be to produce a trial in which it is possible to answer all questions preceding question 40 in the affirmative.

1. Are you convinced that the trial is necessary?
....(Y) (N)
Answer *no* if the trial is a demonstration trial, or if you believe the answer to the question being addressed in the trial is known.

2. Is the trial large enough and the period of treatment and follow-up sufficient to make it likely that the trial will yield fruitful results?
....(Y) (N)

3. Does the trial address a medically relevant question?
....(Y) (N)

4. Is the primary outcome measure a relevant measure of treatment effect?
....(Y) (N)

5. Is there good reason to believe that the test treatment(s) is (are) safe?
....(Y) (N)

Lean toward *no* in the absence of data bearing on safety, especially if the treatments carry risk, as is likely to be the case with most invasive treatments involving surgery and implanted devices and with most forms of treatment involving drugs or biologics.

6. Is there reason to believe that the test treatments will be effective in treating or preventing the condition targeted in the trial?
....(Y) (N)
Lean toward *no* if the only basis for the belief is theoretical, not buttressed by at least observational studies.

7. Is there likely to be a favorable benefit–risk ratio for persons in the trial?
....(Y) (N)

8. Is the risk of harm to persons from the trial minimized?
....(Y) (N)

9. Does your mother stand to benefit from participation?
....(Y) (N)

10. Is there a state of clinical equipoise underlying the treatments being tested?
....(Y) (N)
In answering, remember that clinical equipoise in this context is a *collective* state of legitimate doubt as to choice or proper course of treatment due to absence of agreement among medical experts. Equipoise is considered to exist even if individual persons are certain as to choice or course, so long as, together, they are more or less equally divided. A state of doubt is legitimate only if informed (i.e., based on careful study and review of existing information by the "treating" physicians).

11. Are the study treatments (test and control treatments) compatible with prevailing norms and standards for care and treatment? ....(Y) (N)

Answer *no* if persons enrolled into the trial are denied access to accepted forms of treatment, are likely to receive substandard care, or if the control treatment is considered to be substandard. Note that, in answering, you must decide whether the "prevailing norms and standards for care" are judged on a regional or on a global basis.

12. If the control treatment involves use of a placebo or a nil or null form of treatment, is that treatment consistent with prevailing norms and standards for care and treatment? ....(Y) (N)

Answer *no* if there is a proven accepted mode of treatment. In answering, you must determine your basis for assessing norms and standards. If you believe that norms and standards for care and treatment are global, then the locale of the trial is irrelevant. If you believe that they are regional, then the country or locale of the trial is relevant.

13. If treatments are administered in double-masked fashion, can they be safely administered in that way? ....(Y) (N)

Answer *no* if you believe that the masking increases the risk of harm to your mother, if the protocol fails to allow for physician judgment in regard to whether to continue treatment, or if the protocol places higher value on the importance of adherence to treatment than on patient safety.

14. If the trial is double-masked, do clinic personnel have the means to unmask treatment in the case of medical emergencies? ....(Y) (N)

15. If your mother is masked to treatment, will she be informed of the treatment assignment when she leaves the trial or when the trial is finished?
....(Y) (N)

16. Will your mother be told the results of the trial when it is finished?
....(Y) (N)

17. Is it likely that your mother will be treated with respect by clinic personnel?
....(Y) (N)

18. Will she be treated as an autonomous person?
....(Y) (N)

19. Is subject selection equitable in the trial?
....(Y) (N)
Answer *no* if the trial is designed to exclude a gender group, persons of a particular race or ethnic origin, or persons of a specified age, if the condition being treated in the trial affects both gender groups, is no respecter of race or ethnic origin, or is present in other age groups. Answer *no* also if the trial is designed to concentrate on vulnerable or disadvantaged persons for no apparent reason.

20. Will the information your mother provides and will the data collected on her be kept confidential?
....(Y) (N)

21. Will study personnel respect and protect her privacy?
....(Y) (N)

22. Will your mother be provided with the information necessary for her to make an informed judgment regarding participation?
....(Y) (N)
Answer *no* if you consider information provided in consent form(s) to be inadequate, incomplete, or misleading, or if the reading level is too high.

23. Is the consent process adequate?
....(Y) (N)
Consider answering *no* if consent is not solicited in a quiet, private setting; if you think your mother will feel pressured to make a decision on the spot; if staff do not have the time or patience to answer her questions concerning the trial; or if she does not have time to discuss the pros and cons of participation with family members prior to deciding to enroll.

24. If she agrees to enroll, will she be free to terminate her participation at any time without prejudice?
....(Y) (N)

25. Are investigators in charge of the trial and its conduct?
....(Y) (N)
Answer *no* if investigators cannot modify the protocol without sponsor approval or if a treatment group or the trial cannot be stopped without sponsor approval.

26. Is the study protocol written in such a way that is clear that investigators are obliged to depart from it if doing so is considered to be in the best interest of persons enrolled?
....(Y) (N)

27. Are investigators competent?
....(Y) (N)
Answer *no* if you believe they lack the knowledge, skill, training, or experience necessary for the proper and safe conduct of the trial.

28. Are the investigators trustworthy?
....(Y) (N)

29. Is the data collection schedule reasonable and practical?
....(Y) (N)

30. Are the procedures to which your mother will be exposed necessary and safe?
....(Y) (N)

31. Is the primary analysis by treatment assigned (intention to treat)?
....(Y) (N)
Answer *no* in the absence of statements in the protocol indicating that the primary analysis will be by intention to treat.

32. Are the results of the trial being monitored by a body constituted for that purpose (typically referred to as a data and safety monitoring committee or by other names, such as treatment effects monitoring committee or data monitoring committee)?
....(Y) (N)

33. Is that monitoring body charged with the responsibility for recommending whether the trial should be stopped or altered based on interim looks at study data?
....(Y) (N)

34. Are the analyses presented to that body based on a timely flow of data from collection to analyses and performed by a competent data coordinating center?
....(Y) (N)
Lean toward answering *no* if flow is not designed to be continuous, if the case report form of data flow is employed (i.e., in which forms for a person are submitted for processing as a package at the end of treatment and follow-up), if data entry and processing is

not continuous, or if data analyses are not done by personnel trained for data analyses.

35. Is the monitoring body free of constraint in regard to what it may look at or in how it may look?
....(Y) (N)
Lean toward answering *no* if the body is masked, if it is required to operate under externally imposed stopping rules, or if it is empowered to address only issues of safety.

36. Is there an inalienable link of the monitoring body to study investigators?
....(Y) (N)
Answer *no* if the monitoring body is charged to report to the sponsor and the sponsor has not provided written assurance to investigators that any recommendation for change, regardless of whether supported or opposed by the sponsor, will pass to study investigators in a timely fashion. Answer *yes* if the body reports directly to study leaders or simultaneously to investigators and sponsor.

37. Are investigators free of financial, operational, and philosophical conflicts of interests in regard to the trial?
....(Y) (N)
Answer *no* in the absence of a system, within the trial, for disclosure of conflicts, for reviewing disclosures, and for, when indicated, insulating the trial from persons considered to have conflicts serving to disqualify them from participation or serving to place limits on participation.

38. Are investigators free to publish results from the trial as they deem reasonable and necessary, without fear or prospect of interdiction by sponsors?
....(Y) (N)

Answer *no* if the funding agreement with the sponsor places restrictions or limitations on publication or if the sponsor has right of approval of what or when something is published.

39. Are investigators committed to publishing results of the trial regardless of the nature or direction of the results?
....(Y) (N)
Lean toward answering *no* in the absence of study policy indicating such intent.

40. The Mother Test: *Assuming your mother is eligible and willing to be enrolled into the trial, would you be willing to randomize her to treatment and have her treated and followed as proposed?*
....(Y) (N)

If you answer *yes* to this question and *no* to one or more of the questions above, either you are not as devoted to your mother as you think, or you do not believe that issues addressed in questions for which you answered *no* are important in applying the Mother Test. Explain.

If you answered *no*, even though you answered *yes* to questions 1 through 39, either you do not believe in randomized trials (if so, you should find some other profession), or the list of questions does not cover issues central to your value system. Explain.

If you answered *no* because you answered *no* to one or more of questions 1 through 39, detail the changes or conditions that would have to be satisfied in order for you to allow your mother to enroll into the trial. Explain.

Appendix B

Rating Index for Clinical Trials

Instructions

Step 1: Complete Section A: **Clinical relevance index**. Cumulative scores range from 5 to 21. If the score is high, proceed; if ≤ 10 look for some other trial more relevant to your interest or condition

Step 2: Determine your skepticism level by completing Section B: **Skepticism index**. Keep a running score as you proceed. If at any time it is 30 or higher, your level of skepticism is probably too high for you to have any faith in the results. Try to find another trial yielding a lower skepticism score.

Step 3: Proceed to Section C: **Analysis and discussion confidence index** if skepticism index score is low. Cumulate your score as you proceed. If at any time, the score drops below 15 look for another trial with a higher analysis and discussion index.

Step 4: Section D: **The coup de grâce questions** are the pay dirt section. Believe the results and proceed accordingly if the cumulative score is 20. If it is zero forget it! If it is between zero and 20 proceed with caution.

Note: The weights for responses are arbitrary. If you think the weights should be different you can assign your own.

Score Sum

A. Clinical relevance index

1. Primary outcome measure? (see Chapter 3) ____ ____
   3 Clinical event
   2 Surrogate outcome measure
   1 Change measure
   0 Not specified

2. Clinical relevance of outcome measure to
condition of interest? ____ ____
   3 High
   2 Intermediate
   1 Low

3. Eligibility and exclusion criteria appropriate? ____ ____
   3 Yes
   0 No

4. Eligibility requirements relevant to my condition? ____ ____
   3 Yes
   0 No

5. "Real world" treatment regimen? ____ ____
   3 Closely parallels real world regimen
   2 Modestly parallel to real world regimen
   1 Remotely related to real world regimen

6. Place of conduct? ____ ____
   2 Similar to where I would go for care
   1 Not similar to where I would go for care

7. Period of treatment? ____ ____
   2 Period of treatment sufficient to assess
      safety and efficacy of treatment
   1 Period of treatment too short to be able to
      reliably assess safety and efficacy

Score Sum

8. Period of followup? ____ ____
   2 Period sufficient to assess safety and efficacy of treatment
   1 Period not sufficient to assess safety and efficacy

B. Skepticism index

1. Where published? ____ ____
   30 Self published
   25 Throwaway medical journal
   10 Newspaper/news stand magazine
   5 Book/monograph/meeting proceedings
   5 Medical journal, not NLM-indexed (i.e., not in PubMed)
   0 Medical journal, in PubMed

2. Published in a major, high circulation,
   medical journal? ____ ____
   3 No
   0 Yes

3. Authorship format? (see Chapter 6) ____ ____
   30 No authorship attribution
   15 Byline
   2 Conventional
   1 Modified conventional
   0 Corporate

4. Institutional affiliation of investigators provided? ____ ____
   15 No
   0 Yes

5. Sponsorship? ____ ____
   15 Not stated
   2 Drug company/for profit business
   1 Non profit foundation
   0 NIH/Governmental agency

Score Sum

6. Site of conduct?　　　　　　　　　　　　　　____ ____
    3 Single site (single-center)
    0 Multiple sites (multicenter)

7. Purpose of trial?　　　　　　　　　　　　　____ ____
    15 Not stated/cannot determine
    2 Non-inferiority (to show test treatment not
       worse than comparator treatment)
    2 Equivalence (to show test treatment equivalent
       to comparator treatment)
    0 Superiority (to show test treatment superior
       to comparator treatment)
    2 Other

8. Reason for publication?　　　　　　　　　　　____ ____
    15 Not stated/cannot determine
    5 Interim report (trial still continuing; no
       major change in the study protocol)
    0 Early stop of trial because of evidence of
       benefit or harm (see Chapter 2)
    0 Normal end (trial went to scheduled end)

9. Comparison group?　　　　　　　　　　　　____ ____
    5 None
    5 External/historical control (see Chapter 1)
    0 Internal (concurrently enrolled and followed)

10. Treatment groups?　　　　　　　　　　　　____ ____
    5 One
    0 Two or more (including control treatment)

11. Mode of treatment assignment?
    (see discussion in Chapter 2)　　　　　　　____ ____
    25 Only one treatment group
    25 Patient/physician choice

Score Sum

15 Systematic (e.g., odd days to test treatment;
even days to control treatment)
15 Open "random" (e.g., test treatment if last digit of
hospital record odd; control treatment if even)
5 Concealed "random"; claimed but insufficient detail to determine
0 Concealed random; detailed

12. Primary outcome measure specified? ____ ____
10 No
0 Yes

13. Risk of bias in primary outcome? ____ ____
10 Primary outcome not specified/cannot determine
7 High (unmasked and subjective measure)
3 Low (double masked and subjective measure)
0 Nil (objective measure like death or laboratory test)

14. Masking? ____ ____
2 None
1 Single
0 Double

15. CONSORT-like chart or table giving numbers
enrolled and followed?[3] ____ ____
30 No
0 Yes

16. Rationale for sample size stated? ____ ____
20 No
0 Yes

17. Sample size adequate for conclusions reached? ____ ____
30 No
15 Uncertain
0 Yes

Score Sum

18. Study participants followed regardless of
    compliance to treatment?   ____ ____
    30 No
    15 Uncertain
     0 Yes

19. Analysis limited to "evaluable" patients?   ____ ____
    30 Yes
    15 Uncertain
     0 No

C. Analysis and discussion confidence index

1. All persons assessed for outcome regardless of
   adherence to treatment?   ____ ____
   15 Yes
    0 Cannot determine
   -5 No

2. All outcome events counted from moment of
   enrollment forward in time?   ____ ____
   15 Yes
    0 Cannot determine
   -5 No

3. All persons counted to treatment group to which
   assigned (i.e., ITT)?   ____ ____
   15 Yes
    0 No/Cannot determine

4. Are the conclusions supported by the data?   ____ ____
   15 Yes
    0 No

Score Sum

5. Is the conclusion about a subgroup
   effect or interaction? _____ _____
   15 No
    5 Yes

6. Subgroup analyses to assess homogeneity of
   treatment effect? (see Chapter 17) _____ _____
   15 Yes
    0 No/uncertain

7. Dredged subgroup difference? (see Chapter 17) _____ _____
    15 No
     0 Uncertain
   -10 Yes

8. Is the treatment effect homogeneous across
   subgroups? (see Chapter 17) _____ _____
   10 Yes
    0 No

9. Discussion or presentation of side effect data? _____ _____
   15 Yes
    0 No

10. Are p-values used as indicators of truth?
    (see Chapter 16) _____ _____
    15 No
    -5 Yes

11. Discussion including summary of relevant
    previous studies and trials? _____ _____
    5 Yes
    0 No

Score Sum

12. Discussion of strengths, weakness, and
    limitations of trial?   ____ ____
    5 Yes
   -5 No

D. The coup de grâce questions

  1. Do I trust the investigators?   ____ ____
    5 Yes
    0 No

  2. Do I believe the results?   ____ ____
    5 Yes
    0 No

  3. Do I think the results have been dredged to
     find a "significant" difference?   ____ ____
    5 No
    0 Yes

  4. Do I believe the results are reproducible?   ____ ____
    5 Yes
    0 No

Appendix C

A Patient's Guide for Deciding Whether to Enroll in a Randomized Trial

This guide has three sections and assumes that you or your loved one is eligible for enrollment into the trial in question and that you are at the point of deciding whether you want to enroll.

Section A is designed to plumb your gut instincts regarding the study personnel and whether you trust and respect them. Trust and respect is paramount. If you check "no" for the last question in the section (Question 11), or if you check several other questions "no," you probably should not enroll and not bother with the other two sections of the form.

Assuming things are still a go after completing Section A, complete Section B of the guide. You should know what enrollment entails according to the information provided and the consent form you are expected to sign if you agree to enroll. A "no" to any question indicates that you did not understand the information you were given or that the consent process was inadequate. You should not agree to consent until you can answer all questions in the section in the affirmative.

Once you are able to answer all questions in **Section B** in the affirmative, you are in a position to complete **Section C** of the guide. You should not enroll unless you are able to answer all questions in the affirmative.

A. Ambience index

1. Am I treated with respect by study personnel?..........(Y) (N)
2. Do clinic personnel talk to me as a fellow
   human being?...................................(Y) (N)
3. Are study staff professional and well-trained?...........(Y) (N)
4. Do study personnel treat their fellow colleagues
   with respect?...................................(Y) (N)
5. Did study personnel take time to explain
   the trial to me? ....(Y) (N)
6. Did study personnel answer my questions
   regarding the trial? ....(Y) (N)
7. Was I given ample time to consider my decision?.......(Y) (N)
8. Is the study clinic neat and clean?...................(Y) (N)
9. Is the study clinic located in a place where I feel safe? ...(Y) (N)
10. Did the person who will be treating me talk to me? .....(Y) (N)
11. Do I trust the study head and his or her personnel? .....(Y) (N)

B. Knowledge index

The dialogue with study personnel during the consent process should enable you to answer all questions in this section in the affirmative. If you check "no" for any question, you should not enroll until you can answer in the affirmative.

I have been informed of the following:

1. Why the trial is being done . . . .(Y) (N)
2. Who is sponsoring the trial. . . . .(Y) (N)
3. Who is in charge of the study. . . . .(Y) (N)
4. Who decides how long the trial will run . . . .(Y) (N)
5. The treatments being tested . . . .(Y) (N)
6. The control/comparison treatment . . . .(Y) (N)
7. The length of treatment . . . .(Y) (N)
8. The possible side effects related to treatment . . . .(Y) (N)
9. That the treatment I receive will be chosen by
   the equivalent of a coin toss . . . .(Y) (N)
10. The chance of my receiving the test treatment . . . .(Y) (N)
11. The chance of my receiving the control/
    comparison treatment. . . . .(Y) (N)
12. How many other centers are participating
    in the trial . . . .(Y) (N)
13. Whether I will know the treatment I am on . . . .(Y) (N)
14. Whether my doctor will know
    the treatment I am on. . . . .(Y) (N)
15. If treatments are masked, the purpose
    of the masking. . . . .(Y) (N)
16. How long I am expected to remain
    on treatment . . . .(Y) (N)
17. How long I am expected to remain in the trial . . . .(Y) (N)
18. The clinic visit schedule. . . . .(Y) (N)
19. Where data are processed. . . . .(Y) (N)
20. What happens to my data if I drop out . . . .(Y) (N)
21. Examination and test procedures performed and
    possible risks . . . .(Y) (N)
22. That I can drop out at any time
    without repercussions. . . . .(Y) (N)

C. Willingness index

1. I am willing to accept any of the treatments being tested in the trial. . . . .(Y) (N)
2. I am willing to have my treatment chosen by the equivalent of a coin toss.. . . . .(Y) (N)
3. I believe the prospect of benefit outweighs the risk of harm if I enroll. . . . .(Y) (N)
4. I believe the care I will receive will be at least as good as that which I would receive if I do not enroll. . . . .(Y) (N)
5. I believe the trial will produce useful results. . . . .(Y) (N)
6. I believe investigators will publish results from the trial regardless of how it turns out. . . . .(Y) (N)
7. I believe the trial is big enough to produce a useful result.. . . . .(Y) (N)
8. I believe the trial is ethically designed and will be ethically conducted. . . . .(Y) (N)
9. I believe I can stick to the clinic visit schedule outlined. . . . .(Y) (N)
10. I intend to stay in the trial regardless of my treatment assignment and schedule. . . . .(Y) (N)
11. I am comfortable that my data will be kept confidential. . . . .(Y) (N)
12. I answered question 40 on the Mother Test in the affirmative. . . . .(Y) (N)

Appendix D

Abbreviations

ACTG	AIDS Clinical Trials Group
ACTH	adrenocorticotropic hormone
ADA	American Diabetes Association
AE	adverse event
Ant	antonym
BMD	bone mineral density
BMJ	*British Medical Journal*
CC	coordinating center
CCD	Committee for the Care of the Diabetic
CDC	Centers for Disease Control and Prevention
CDER	Center for Drug Evaluation and Research
CDP	Coronary Drug Project
CHD	coronary heart disease
CI	confidence interval
CMS	Centers for Medicare & Medicaid Services
CONSORT	Consolidated Standards of Reporting Trials
CRF	case report form
CRO	contract research organization
CT	clinical trial
CV	cardiovascular; curriculum vitae

DHHS	Department of Health and Human Services
DMC	data monitoring committee
DSMB	data and safety monitoring board
DSMC	data and safety monitoring committee
EC	executive committee
FDA	Food and Drug Administration
FOIA	Freedom of Information Act
FWA	federalwide assurance
FY	fiscal year
GRASE	generally recognized as safe and effective
HAART	highly active antiretroviral therapy
HDFP	Hypertension Detection and Followup Program
HIPAA	Health Insurance Portability and Accountability Act
HIV	human immunodeficiency virus
HPT	Hypertension Prevention Trial
ICMJE	International Committee of Medical Journal Editors
IND	Investigational New Drug
INDA	Investigational New Drug Application
IRB	institutional review board
ITT	intention to treat
JAMA	*Journal of the American Medical Association*
MI	myocardial infarction
MOO, MoO, MOP, MOp	manual of operations
MRFIT	Multiple Risk Factor Intervention Trial
NDA	New Drug Application
NEJM	*New England Journal of Medicine*
NIH	National Institutes of Health
NLM	National Library of Medicine
NSABP	National Surgical Adjuvant and Bowel Project
NSAIDs	nonsteroidal anti-inflammatory drugs
OHRP	Office for Human Research Protections
OMB	Office of Management and Budget
ONJ	osteonecrosis of the jaw
OPRR	Office for Protection from Research Risks

ORI	Office of Research Integrity
ORWH	Office of Research on Women's Health
OSI	Office of Scientific Integrity
PAA	per assignment analysis
PDR	*Physicians' Desk Reference*
PHS	Public Health Service
PI	principal investigator
PLoS	Public Library of Science
PPA	per protocol analysis
PPM	policy and procedure memorandum
[ptyp], [pt]	publication type
RCT	randomized clinical trial, randomized control trial, randomized controlled trial
RFA	request for application
RFP	request for proposal
Rz	randomized
rt	related term
Rz CT, RzCT	randomized clinical trial, randomized controlled trial
SC	steering committee
TEMC	treatment effects monitoring committee
UGDP	University Group Diabetes Program
USPHS	United States Public Health Service
USPSTF	U.S. Preventive Services Task Force
WHA	World Health Association
WHI	Women's Health Initiative

References

1. **ADAPT** Research Group. Naproxen and celecoxib do not prevent AD in early results from a randomized controlled trial. *Neurology.* 2007;68;1800–1808.

    ch3, ch4, ch14

2. **ADAPT** Research Group. Cardiovascular and cerebrovascular results from the randomized, controlled Alzheimer's Disease Anti-inflammatory Prevention Trial (ADAPT). *PLoS Clin Trials.* 2006; 1(7):e33.

    ch13, ch14

3. **Altman** DG, Schulz KF, Moher D, Egger M, Davidoff F, Elbourne D, Gøtzsche PC, Lang T: The revised CONSORT statement for reporting randomized trials: Explanation and elaboration. *Ann Intern Med.* 2001; 134: 663–694.

    ch13, ch15, appB

4. **Amberson** JB, Jr., McMahon BT, Pinner M. A clinical trial of sanocrysin in pulmonary tuberculosis. *Am Rev Tuberc.* 1931; 24:401–435.

    ch1

5. **American Bible Society.** *The Holy Bible: Old and New Testaments.* King James Version (1611). New York: 1816.

    ch1

6. **Angell** M. Industry-sponsored clinical research: A broken system. *JAMA.* 2008; 300:1069–1071.

    ch11

7. **Angell** M. Investigators' responsibility for human subjects in developing countries. *N Engl J Med.* 2000; 342:967–969.

    ch11

8. **Antithrombotic Trialists' Collaboration**. Collaborative meta-analysis of randomised trials of antiplatelet therapy for prevention of death, myocardial infarction, and stroke in high risk patients. *BMJ*. **2002**; 324:71–86.

ch18, ch19

9. **Antiplatelet Trialists' Collaboration**. Collaborative overview of randomized trials of antiplatelet therapy. I: Prevention of death, myocardial infarction, and stroke by prolonged antiplatelet therapy in various categories of patients. *BMJ*. **1994**; 308:81–106.

ch19

10. **Antman** EM, Lau J, Kupeinick B, Mosteller F, Chalmers TC. A comparison of results of meta-analyses of randomized control trials and recommendations of clinical experts. *JAMA*. **1992**; 268:240–248.

ch18

11. **Bailey** KR. Detecting fabrication of data in a multicenter collaborative animal study. *Control Clin Trials*. **1991**; 12:741–752.

ch10

12. **Baron** J. The life of Edward Jenner: With illustrations of his doctrines and selections from his correspondence (book review). *Br Foreign Med Rev*. **1838**; 6:477–497.

ch22

13. **Bartolucci** AA, Howard G. Meta-analysis of data from the six primary prevention trials of cardiovascular events using aspirin. *Am J Cardiol*. **2006**; 98:746–750.

ch19

14. **Beecher** HK. Ethics and clinical research. *N Engl J Med*. **1966**; 274: 1354–1360.

ch8

15. **Begg** C, Cho M, Eastwood S, Horton R, Moher D, Olkin I, Pitkin R, Rennie D, Schultz KF, Simel D, Stroup DF. Improving the quality of reporting of randomized controlled trials: The CONSORT statement. *JAMA*. **1996**; 276:637–639.

ch9

16. **Berger** JS, Roncaglioni MC, Avanzini F, Pangrazzi I, Tognoni G, Brown DL. Aspirin for the primary prevention of cardiovascular events in women and men: A sex-specific meta-analysis of randomized controlled trials. *JAMA*. **2006**; 295:306–313.

ch19

17. *Black's Law Dictionary*. St. Paul, MN: West Publishing Company, **1990**.

ch10

18. **Box** JF. RA Fisher and the design of experiments, 1922–1926. *Am Statistician*. **1980**; 34:1–7.

ch1

19. **Broad** WJ.: U.S. to penalize heart researchers on fraudulent project at Harvard. *New York Times.* 16 February 1983.

ch10

20. **Brookmeyer** R, Gray S, Kawas C. Projections of Alzheimer's disease in the United States and the public health impact of delaying disease onset. *Am J Pub Health.* 1998; 88:1337–1342.

ch12

21. **Canner** PL. Aspirin in coronary heart disease: Comparison of six clinical trials. *Isr J Med Sci.* 1983; 19:413–423.

ch19

22. **Childhood Asthma Management Program Research Group**. The Childhood Asthma Management Program (CAMP): Design, rationale, and methods. *Control Clin Trials.* 1999; 20:91–120.

ch4

23. **Collins** JF, Garg R, Koon KT, Williford WO, Howell CL on behalf of DIG Investigators. The role of the data coordinating center in the IRB review and approval process: The DIG trial experience. *Control Clin Trials.* 2003; 24:306S–315S.

ch8

24. **Colsky** J. Clinical investigator: The clinical investigator and evaluation of new drugs. *Am J Hosp Pharm.* 1963; 20:517–519.

ch1

25. **Connolly** HM, Crary JL, McGoon MD, Hensrud DD, Edwards BS, Edwards WD, Schaff HV. Valvular heart disease associated with fenfluramine-phentermine. *N Engl J Med.* 1997; 337:581–588.

ch24

26. **Connor** EM, Sperling RS, Gelber R, Kiselev P, Scott G, O'Sullivan MJ, VanDyke R, Bey M, Shearer W, Jacobson RL, Jimenez E, O'Neill E, Bazin B, Delfraissy J-F, Culnane M, Coombs R, Elkins M, Moye J, Stratton P, Balsley J., for the Pediatric AIDS Clinical Trials Group Protocol 076 Study Group. Reduction of maternal-infant transmission of human immuno-deficiency virus type 1 with zidovudine treatment. *N Engl J Med.* 1994; 331:1173–1180.

ch11, ch19

27. **Cornfield** J. Recent methodological contributions to clinical trials. *Am J Epidemiol.* 1976; 104:408–421.

ch11, ch17

28. **Cornfield** J. Design of clinical trials. In Goldstein M, ed., *Research Status of Spinal Manipulative Therapy,* pp. 303–306. Monograph no. 15. Bethesda, MD: National Institute of Neurological and Communicative Disorders and Stroke, 1975.

ch15

29. **Coronary Drug Project Research Group**. Clofibrate and niacin in coronary heart disease. *JAMA*. **1975**; 231:360–381.

ch4

30. **Coronary Drug Project Research Group**. The Coronary Drug Project: Design, methods, and baseline results. *Circulation*. **1973**; 47(Suppl I):I-1–I-50.

ch5, ch16

31. **Couzin** J. Drug testing: Massive trial of Celebrex seeks to settle safety concerns. *Science*. **2005**; 310:1890–1891.

ch19

32. **Creighton** C. *A history of epidemics in Britain: From the extinction of plague to the present time* (vol. II). Cambridge: The University Press, **1894**.

ch22

33. **DeAngelis** CD, Fontanarosa PB. Impugning the integrity of medical science: The adverse effects of industry influence. *JAMA*. **2008**; 299:1833–1835.

ch6, ch13

34. **DeAngelis** CD, Drazen JM, Frizelle FA, Haug C, Hoey J, Horton R, Kotzin S, Laine C, Marusic A, Overbeke AJPM, Schroeder TV, Sox HC, Van Der Weyden MB: Clinical trial registration: A statement from the International Committee of Medical Journal Editors. *JAMA*. **2004**; 292: 1363–1364.

ch9

35. **Department of Health and Human Services**. Public Health Services policies on research misconduct; 42 CFR Parts 50 and 93. *Federal Register*. **2005**; 70:28370–28400.

ch10

36. **Dieckmann** WJ, Davis ME, Rynkiewicz LM, Pottinger RE. Does the administration of diethylstilbestrol during pregnancy have therapeutic value?. *Am J Obst Gynecol*. **1953**; 66:1062–1081.

ch24

37. **Diehl** HS, Baker AB, Cowan DW. Cold vaccines: An evaluation based on a controlled study *JAMA*. **1938**; 111:1168–1173.

ch1

38. **Digitalis Investigation Group**. The effect of digoxin on mortality and morbidity in patients with heart failure. *N Engl J Med*. **1997**; 336:525–533.

ch6, ch8

39. **Drummond** JC, Wilbraham A. *The Englishman's food: A history of five centuries of English diet*. London: Jonathan Cape, **1940**.

ch1

40. **Fenner** F, Henderson DA, Arita I, Landyi ID. *Smallpox and its eradication*. Geneva: World Health Organization, **1988**.

ch22

41. Fergusson D, Glass KC, Hutton B, Shapiro S. Randomized controlled trials of aprotinin in cardiac surgery: Could clinical equipoise have stopped the bleeding? *Clin Trials.* 2005; 2:218–232.

ch19

42. Fisher B, Anderson S, Redmond CK, Wolmark N, Wickerham DL. Reanalysis and results after 12 years of follow-up in a randomized clinical trial comparing total mastectomy with lumpectomy with or without radiation in the treatment of breast cancer. *N Engl J Med.* 1995; 333:1456–1451.

ch10

43. Fisher B, Bauer M, Margolese R, Poisson R, Pilch Y, Redmond C, Fisher E, Wolmark N, Deutsch M, Montague E, et al: Five-year results of a randomized clinical trial comparing total mastectomy and segmental mastectomy with or without radiation in the treatment of breast cancer. *N Engl J Med.* 1985; 312:665–73.

ch10

44. Fisher RA. *Statistical methods and scientific inference* (3rd edition). New York: Hafner Press, Macmillan Publishing Co., 1973.

ch1

45. Fisher RA. The arrangement of field experiments. *J Ministry Agric Great Britain.* 1926; 33:503–513.

ch1

46. Fisher RA, MacKenzie WA. Studies in crop variation: II. The manurial response of different potato varieties. *J Agric Sci.* 1923; 13:311–320.

ch1

47. Food and Drug Administration. Procedural and interpretative regulations: Investigational use. *Federal Register.* January 8, 1963; 28:179–182.

ch1

48. Fost N, Levine RJ. The dysregulation of human subjects research. *JAMA.* 2008; 298:2196–2198.

ch11

49. Francis T, Korns RF, Voigt RB, Boisen M, Hemphill FM, Napier JA, Tolchinsky E. An evaluation of the 1954 poliomyelitis vaccine trial: Summary report. *Am J Public Health.* 1955; 45(Part II, May Suppl):1–51.

ch1

50. Freedman B. Equipoise and the ethics of clinical research. *N Engl J Med.* 1987; 317:141–145.

ch8

51. Freedman LS, Simon R, Foulkes MA, Friedman L, Geller NL, Gordon DJ, Mowery R. Inclusion of women and minorities in clinical trials and the NIH Revitalization Act of 1993—The perspective of NIH clinical trialists (with discussion and response). *Control Clin Trials.* 1995;16:277–312.

ch11

52. **Freis** ED. Historical development of antihypertensive treatment. In Laragh JH, Brenner BM, eds., *Hypertension pathophysiology, diagnosis, and management*, 2nd ed., Chapter 164, pp. 2741–2751. New York: Raven Press, 1995.

ch19

53. **Glass** GV. Primary, secondary and meta-analysis of research. *Educational Researcher.* 1976; 5:3–8.

ch18

54. **Goodman** SN. Toward evidence-based medical statistics. 1: The p value fallacy. *Ann Intern Med.* 1995; 130:995–1004.

ch16

55. **Guay** LA, Musoke P, Fleming T, Bagenda D, Allen M, Nakabito C, Sherman J, Bakaki P, Ducar C, Deseyve M, Emel L, Mirochnick M, Fowler MG, Mofenson L, Miotti P, Dransfield K, Bray D, Mmiro F, Jacksom JB: Intrapartum and neonatal single-dose nevirapine with zidovudine for prevention of mother-to-child transmission of HIV-1 in Kampala, Uganda: HIVNET 012 randomized trial. *Lancet* 1999; 354:795–802.

ch11

56. **Hayes** SN, Redberg RF. Dispelling the myths: Calling for sex-specific reporting of trials results. *Mayo Clin Proc.* 2008; 83:523–525.

ch8

57. **Haygarth** J. *Of the imagination, as a cause and as a cure of disorders of the body: Exemplified by fictitious tractors, and epidemical convulsions.* Bath: R Cruttwell, 1800.

ch2

58. **Herbst** AL, Scully RE. Adenocarcinoma of the vagina in adolescence. A report of 7 cases including 6 clear-cell carcinomas (so-called mesonephromas). *Cancer.* 1970; 25:745–757.

ch24

59. **Hill** AB. *Statistical methods in clinical and preventive medicine.* New York: Oxford University Press, 1962.

ch1

60. **Huff** D. *How to lie with statistics.* Illustrated, I Geis. New York: Norton, 1954.

ch13

61. **Hypertension Detection and Follow-Up Program Cooperative Group**. Five-year findings of the Hypertension Detection and Follow-Up Program: I. Reduction in mortality of persons with high blood pressure, including mild hypertension. *JAMA.* 1979a; 242:2562–2571.

ch1

62. **Hypertension Detection and Follow-up Program**. Therapeutic control of blood pressure in the Hypertension Detection and Follow-up Program. *Prev Med.* 1979; 8:2–13.

ch13

63. **Hypertension Prevention Trial Research Group**, C Meinert, J Tonascia, S Tonasica, eds. The Hypertension Prevention Trial (HPT): Design, methods, and baseline results. *Control Clin Trials.* 1989; 10 (Suppl):1S–17S.

ch10

64. **Ibarreta** D, Swan SH: The DES story: Long-term consequences of prenatal exposure. In Harremoës P, Gee D, MacGarvin M, Stirling A, Keys J, Wynne B, Vaz SG, eds. *Late lessons from early warnings: The precautionary principle 1896–2000.* Chapter 8, pp. 84–91. Copenhagen: European Environment Agency, 2001.

ch24

65. **International Committee of Medical Journal Editors**. Uniform requirements for manuscripts submitted to biomedical journals. *N Engl J Med.* 1997; 336:309–315.

ch6

66. **Jenner** E. *An inquiry into the causes and effects of the variolae vaccine.* London: Sampson Low, 1798.

ch22

67. **Johnson** S. *A dictionary of the English language.* (2 vols.). Printed by W Strahan, for J and P Knapton; T and T Longman; C Hitch and L Hawes; A Millar; and R and J Dodsley, 1755.

ch2

68. **Kassirer** JP, Angell M. On authorship and acknowledgments. *N Engl J Med.* 1991; 325:1510–1512.

ch6

69. **Kelsey** FO. Government: The Kefauver-Harris Amendments and investigational drugs. *Am J Hosp Pharm.* 1963; 20:515–517.

ch1

70. **Kluger** J. *Splendid solution: Jonas Salk and the conquest of polio.* New York: Penguin Group (USA), 2005.

ch22

71. **Last** JM. *A dictionary of epidemiology* (4th edition). New York: Oxford University Press, 2001.

ch16

72. **Levine** RJ. *Ethics and regulation of clinical research* (2nd edition). New Haven: Yale University Press, 1988.

ch8, ch9

73. **Lewis** S, Clarke M.: Forest plots: Trying to see the wood and the trees. *BMJ.* 2001;322:1479–1480.

ch18

74. **Lind** J. *A treatise of the scurvy* (reprinted in Lind's Treatise on scurvy, edited by CP Stewart, D Guthrie, Edinburgh University Press, Edinburgh, 1953). Edinburgh: Sands, Murray, Cochran, 1753.

ch1

75. **MacLean** C, Newberry S, Maglione M, McMahon M, Ranganath V, Suttorp M, et al. Systematic review: Comparative effectiveness of treatments to prevent fractures in men and women with low bone density or osteoporosis. *Ann Intern Med.* **2008**; 148:197–213.

ch18

76. **Markel** H. April 12, 1955 – Tommy Francis and the Salk Vaccine. *N Engl J Med.* **2005**; 352:1408–1410.

ch1

77. **Medical Research Council.** Streptomycin treatment of pulmonary tuberculosis: A Medical Research Council investigation. *Br Med J.* **1948**; 2:769–782.

ch1

78. **Medical Research Council.** Clinical trials of new remedies (annotations). *Lancet.* **1931**; 2:304.

ch1

79. **Meinert** C, Gilpin AK, Ünalp A, Dawson C. Gender representation in trials. *Control Clin Trials.* **2000**; 21:462–475.

ch11

80. **Meinert** CL. *Controlled Clinical Trials* (the journal). *Encyclopedia of biostatistics,* vol. 1, pp. 929–931. Chichester, UK: John Wiley & Sons,1998.

ch1

81. **Meinert** CL. Beyond CONSORT: Need for improved reporting standards for clinical trials. *JAMA.* **1998**; 279:1487–1489.

ch9

82. **Meinert** CL. Masked monitoring in clinical trials—Blind stupidity?. *N Engl J Med.* **1998**; 338:1381–1382.

ch11, ch23, ch24

83. **Meinert** CL. *Clinical trials dictionary: Terminology and usage recommendations.* Baltimore, MD: The Johns Hopkins Center for Clinical Trials, **1996**.

v, ch2, ch10

84. **Meinert** CL, Tonascia S. *Clinical trials:Design, conduct, and analysis.* New York: Oxford University Press, **1986**.

v, ix, ch14, ch15

85. **Miller** PD, Epstein S, Sedarati F, Reginster JY. Once-monthly oral ibandronate compared with weekly oral alendronate in postmenopausal osteoporosis: Results from the head-to-head MOTION study. *Curr Med Res Opin.* **2008**; 1:207–213.

ch18

86. **Mills** JL. Data torturing. *N Engl J Med.* **1993**; 329:1196–1199.

ch16

87. **Moher** D. CONSORT: An evolving tool to help improve the quality of reports of randomized controlled trials. *JAMA.* **1998**; 279:1489–1491.

ch9

88. **Mount** FW, Ferebee SH. Control study of comparative efficacy of isoniazid, streptomycin-isoniazid, and streptomycin-para-aminosalicylic acid in pulmonary tuberculosis therapy: II. Report on twenty-week observations on 390 patients with streptomycin-susceptible infections. *Am Rev Tuberc.* 1953a; 67:108–113.

ch1

89. **Mount** FW, Ferebee SH. Control study of comparative efficacy of isoniazid, streptomycin-isoniazid, and streptomycin-para-aminosalicylic acid in pulmonary tuberculosis therapy: III. Report on twenty-eight-week observations on 649 patients with streptomycin-susceptible infections. *Am Rev Tuberc.* 1953b; 67:539–543.

ch1

90. **Mount** FW, Ferebee SH. Control study of comparative efficacy of isoniazid, streptomycin-isoniazid, and streptomycin-para-aminosalicylic acid in pulmonary tuberculosis therapy: I. Report on twelve-week observations on 526 patients. *Am Rev Tuberc.* 1952; 66:632–635.

ch1

91. **Multiple Risk Factor Intervention Trial Research Group.** Statistical design considerations in the NHLI Multiple Risk Factor Intervention Trial (MRFIT). *J Chronic Dis.* 1977; 30:261–275.

ch1

92. **Murray** JAH, Bradley H, Craigie WA, Onion CT, eds. *The Oxford English dictionary:A new English dictionary on historical principles* (13 vols.). Oxford: Clarendon Press, 1970.

ch10

93. **National Commission for the Protection of Human Subjects of Biomedical and Behavioral Research.** *The Belmont Report: Ethical principles and guidelines for the protection of human subjects of research.* No. 1983–381–132:3205. Washington, DC: US Government Printing Office, 1979.

ch8, ch23

94. **U.S. Congress.** *National Institutes of Health Revitalization Act of 1993.* §131, Pub L No 103–43, 107 Stat 133 (codified at 42 USC §289a-2).

ch7

95. **National Institutes of Health Department of Health and Human Services:** NIH Guidelines on the inclusion of women and minorities as subjects in clinical research. *Federal Register.* March 28 1994; 59:14508–14513.

ch7

96. **National Institutes of Health.** *NIH Almanac.* Publ. no. 81–5. Bethesda, MD: Division of Public Information, 1981b.

ch1

97. **Neaton** JD, Bartsch GE, Broste SK, Cohen JD, Simon NM, for the MRFIT Research Group. A case of data alteration in the Multiple Risk Factor Intervention Trials (MRFIT). *Control Clin Trials.* **1991**; 12:731–740.

ch10

98. **Nissen** SE, Wolski K. Effect of rosiglitazone on the risk of myocardial infraction and death from cardiovascular causes. *N Engl J Med.* **2007**; 356:2457–2471.

ch18

99. **O'Brien** PC. Data and safety monitoring. In *Encyclopedia of biostatistics,* vol. 2, pp. 1058–1066. Chichester: John Wiley & Sons, **1998**.

ch23

100. **Office for Protection from Research Risks.** *Code of Federal Regulations, Title 45: Public Welfare, Part 46: Protection of Human Subjects.* Bethesda, MD: Department of Health and Human Services, National Institutes of Health, revised 18 June **1991**.

ch9, ch23

101. **Ogawa** H, Nakayama M, Morimoto T, Uemura S, Kanauchi M, Doi N, Jinnouchi H, Sugiyama S, Saito Y, for the Japanese Primary Prevention of Atherosclerosis With Aspirin for Diabetes (JPAD) Trial Investigators. Low-dose aspirin for primary prevention of atherosclerotic events in patients with type 2 diabetes: A randomized controlled trial. *JAMA.* **2008**; 300: 2134–2141.

ch19

102. **Packard** FR. *Life and times of Ambroise Paré, 1510–1590.* New York: Paul B Hoeber, **1921**.

ch19

103. **Patulin Clinical Trials Committee** (of the Medical Research Council). Clinical trial of Patulin in the common cold. *Lancet.* **1944**; 2:373–375.

ch1

104. **Peto** R, Collins R, Sackett D, Darbyshire J, Babiker A, Buyse M, Stewart H, Baum M, Goldhirsh A, Bonadonna G, Valagussa P, Rutqvist L, Elbourne D, Davies C, Dalesio O, Parmar M, Hill C, Clarke M, Gray R, Doll R: The trials of Dr. Bernard Fisher: A European perspective on an American episode. *Control Clin Trials.* **1997**; 18:1–13.

ch10

105. **Physicians' Health Study Research Group Steering Committee.** Preliminary report: Findings from the aspirin component of the ongoing Physicians' Health Study. *N Engl J Med.* **1988**; 318:262–264.

ch1, ch23

106. **Polman** CH, O'Connor PW, Havrdova E, Hutchinson M, Kappos L, Miller DH, Phillips T, Lubin FD, Giovannoni G, Wajgt A, Toal M, Lynn F, Panzara MA, Sandrock AW for the AFIRM Investigators. A randomized, placebo-controlled

trial of natalizumab for relapsing multiple sclerosis. N Engl J Med. 2006; 354:899–910.

ch13

107. **Pruitt** Jr. BA, Pruitt JH, Davis JH. Chapter 1, pp. 1–19. In Moore EE, Felficiano DV, Mattox KL, eds., Trauma (5th edition). New York: McGraw-Hill Professional, 2003.

ch19

108. **Rennie** D. Clinical trial misconduct. In Wiley encyclopedia of clinical trials. New York: John Wiley & Sons, 2007. Online at http://mrw.interscience.wiley.com/emrw/9780471462422/wect/article/eoct060/current/pdf

ch10

109. **Rennie** D. How to report randomized controlled trials: The CONSORT statement. JAMA. 1996; 276:649.

ch9

110. **Ries** LAG. Childhood cancer mortality. In Ries LAG, Smith MA, Gurney JG, Linet M, Tamra T, Young JL, Bunin GR, eds. Cancer incidence and survival among children and adolescents: United States SEER program: 1975–1995, pp. 165–170. SEER Monograph, Pub. No. 99–4649. Bethesda, MD: National Cancer Institute, 1999.

ch22

111. **Rheumatic Fever Working Party of the Medical Research Council of Great Britain and the Subcommittee of Principal Investigators of the American Council of Rheumatic Fever and Congenital Heart Disease, American Heart Association.** The evolution of rheumatic heart disease in children: Five year report of a cooperative clinical trial of ACTH, cortisone and aspirin. Circulation. 1960; 22:503–515.

ch1

112. **Robinson** D, Shettles L. The use of diethylstilbestrol in threatened abortion. Am J Obstet Gynecol. 1952; 63:1330–1333.

ch24

113. **Savulescu** J, Chalmers I, Blunt J. Are research ethics committees behaving unethically? Some suggestions for improving performance and accountability. Br Med J. 1996; 313:1390–1393.

ch19

114. **Shuster** E. Fifty years later: The significance of the Nüremberg Code. N Engl J Med. 1997; 337:1436–1440.

ch8

115. **Stampfer** MJ, Colditz GA. Estrogen replacement therapy and coronary heart disease: A quantitative assessment of the epidemiological data. Prev Med. 1991; 20:47–63.

ch1

116. **Titus** SL, Rhoades LJ. Repairing research integrity. *Nature.* **2008**; 453: 980–982.

ch10, ch11

117. **Thomas** KJ, MacPherson H, Trope L, Brazier J, Fitter M, Campbell MJ, Roman M, Walters SJ, Nicholl J: Randomised controlled trial of a short course of traditional acupuncture compared with usual care for persistent non-specific low back pain. *BMJ.* **2006**; 333:623.

ch13

118. **Tucker** WB. The evolution of the cooperative studies in the chemotherapy of tuberculosis of the Veterans Administration and Armed Forces of the USA: An account of the evolving education of the physician in clinical pharmacology. *Adv Tuberc Res.* **1960**; 10:1–68.

ch1

119. **United States Congress** (103rd; 1st session). *NIH Revitalization Act of 1993, 42 USC § 131 (1993); Clinical Research Equity Regarding Women and Minorities; Part I: Women and Minorities as Subjects in Clinical Research.* **1993**.

ch11

120. **United States Congress** (87th): *Drug Amendments of 1962*, Public Law 87–781, S 1522. Washington, DC, Oct 10, **1962**.

ch1

121. **United States Supreme Court**. *Forsham et al. versus Harris, Secretary of Health, Education and Welfare, et al.* Certiorari to the United States Court of Appeals for the District of Columbia Circuit. No. 78–1118, argued Oct 31, 1979, decided March 3, **1980**.

ch15, ch23

122. **University Group Diabetes Program Research Group**. Effects of hypoglyce-mic agents on vascular complications in patients with adult-onset diabetes: VIII. Evaluation of insulin therapy: Final report. *Diabetes.* **1982**; 31 (Suppl 5):1–81.

ch4

123. **University Group Diabetes Program Research Group**. Effects of hypoglyce-mic agents on vascular complications in patients with adult-onset diabetes: VII. Mortality and selected nonfatal events with insulin treatment. *JAMA.* **1978**;240:37–42.

ch1, ch3

124. **University Group Diabetes Program Research Group**. A Study of the effects of hypoglycemic agents on vascular complications in patients with adult-onset diabetes:V. Evaluation of Phenformin therapy. *Diabetes.* **1975**; 24 (Suppl 1): 65–184.

ch4

125. University Group Diabetes Program Research Group. A study of the effects of hypoglycemic agents on vascular complications in patients with adult-onset diabetes: I. Design, methods, and baseline characteristics. *Diabetes*. 1970; 19(Suppl 2):747–783.

ix, ch3, ch4, ch19

126. University Group Diabetes Program Research Group. A study of the effects of hypoglycemic agents on vascular complications in patients with adult-onset diabetes: II. Mortality results. *Diabetes* 1970; 19(Suppl 2):785–830.

ch1, ch19

127. U.S. Preventive Services Task Force. Aspirin for the Primary Prevention of Cardiovascular Events: Recommendation and Rationale. *Ann Inter Med.* 2002; 136:157–160.

ch19

128. Vuthipongse P, Bhadrakom C, Chaisilwattana P, Roongpisuthipong A, Chalermchokcharoenkit A Chearskul S, Wanprapa N, Chokephaibulkit K, Tuchipda M, Wasi C, Chuachoowong R, Siriwasin W, Chinayon P, Asavapiriyanont S, Chotpitayasunondh T, Waranawat N, Sangtaweesin V, Horpaopan S, Queen Sirikit: Administration of zidovudine during late pregnancy and delivery to prevent perinatal HIV transmission – Thailand, 1996–1998. *MMWR*. 1998; 47:151–153.

ch11

129. Wells GA, Cranney A, Peterson J, Boucher M, Shea B, Robinson V, Coyle D, Tugwell P: Alendronate for the primary and secondary prevention of osteoporotic fractures in postmenopausal women. *Cochrane Database Syst Rev*. 2008 Jan 23.

ch18

130. Writing Group for the Women's Health Initiative Investigators. Risks and benefits of estrogen plus progestin in healthy postmenopausal women: Principal results from the Women's Health Initiative Randomized Controlled Trial. *JAMA*. 2002; 288:321–333.

ch1, ch3, ch15

131. Yusuf S, Wittes J, Probstfield J, Tyroler HA. Analysis and interpretation of treatment effects in subgroups of patients in randomized clinical trials. *JAMA*. 1991; 266:93–98.

ch17

132. Zarin DA, Ide NC, Tse T, Harlan WR, West JC, Lindberg DA. Issues in the registration of clinical trials. *JAMA*. 2007; 297:2112–2120.

ch9

Author Index

Subject Index

Antithrombotic Trialists' Collaboration, 161, 170
approved label, 21
Aristotle, 37
aspirin, 170–72
authorship. *See also* credits
  certifying, 49
  group, 54
  in multicenter trials, 52–55
  order of, 53–54, 53n1
Avandia, 160, 163–64

back dating, 86
  in SOCA, 88
baseline, 17
  randomization and differences of, 139–40
  of treatment groups, 98
baseline comparability, 14
baseline data, 17
basic reference manuals, 181
Baum, L. Frank, 189
Bayan, Rick, 189
Bayesian, 137, 141. *See also* frequentist; likelihoodist
Bayesian analysis, 141. *See also* frequentist analysis; likelihoodist
Belmont Report, 71, 75, 206, 208, 212
beneficence, principle of, 71
bias, 14
  detecting, 116
  publication, 27, 96
Bierce, Ambrose, 189
biostatistics, 137–50
  textbooks on, 177–78
blackout modes of operation, 74
Black's Law Dictionary, 86
blind(ing)
  identifying, 115
  mask compared to, 18–19

blind/mask. *See* double mask/blind; mask(ing); single mask/blind
blocking
  randomization and, 15
  stratification compared to, 208
BMD. *See* bone mineral density
BMJ. *See British Medical Journal*
bone mineral density (BMD), 159
Boniva (ibandronate), 162–63
The Boy Who Cried Wolf (Aesop), 190
British Medical Journal (BMJ), 41, 42t
Butler, Ellis Parker, 125n1, 189–90

CAMP. *See* Childhood Asthma Management Program
Campbell, Joseph, 91
cancer, 194
Carroll, Robert T., 189
CCD. *See* Committee for the Care of the Diabetic
CDP. *See* Coronary Drug Project
Celebrex, 169
celecoxib (Celebrex), 169
censor/censoring, 141–42
CFR. *See* Code of Federal Regulations
Chicken Little, 188
Childhood Asthma Management Program (CAMP), 33t
Churchill, Winston, 77, 125
clever critics, 119
clinical, 1, 21–22
  relevance, 29
clinical equipoise, 73, 214
Clinical Relevance Index, 129–30
clinical trials, 21–22. *See also* trials; specific types
  drug companies performing, 96
  everyday usage of, 2
  by gender, 63, 64t
  language of, 11–22
  NLM definition of, 7–8, 207